AF249129

Reflections of the Heart

Stories from a Cosmetic Surgeon's Practice

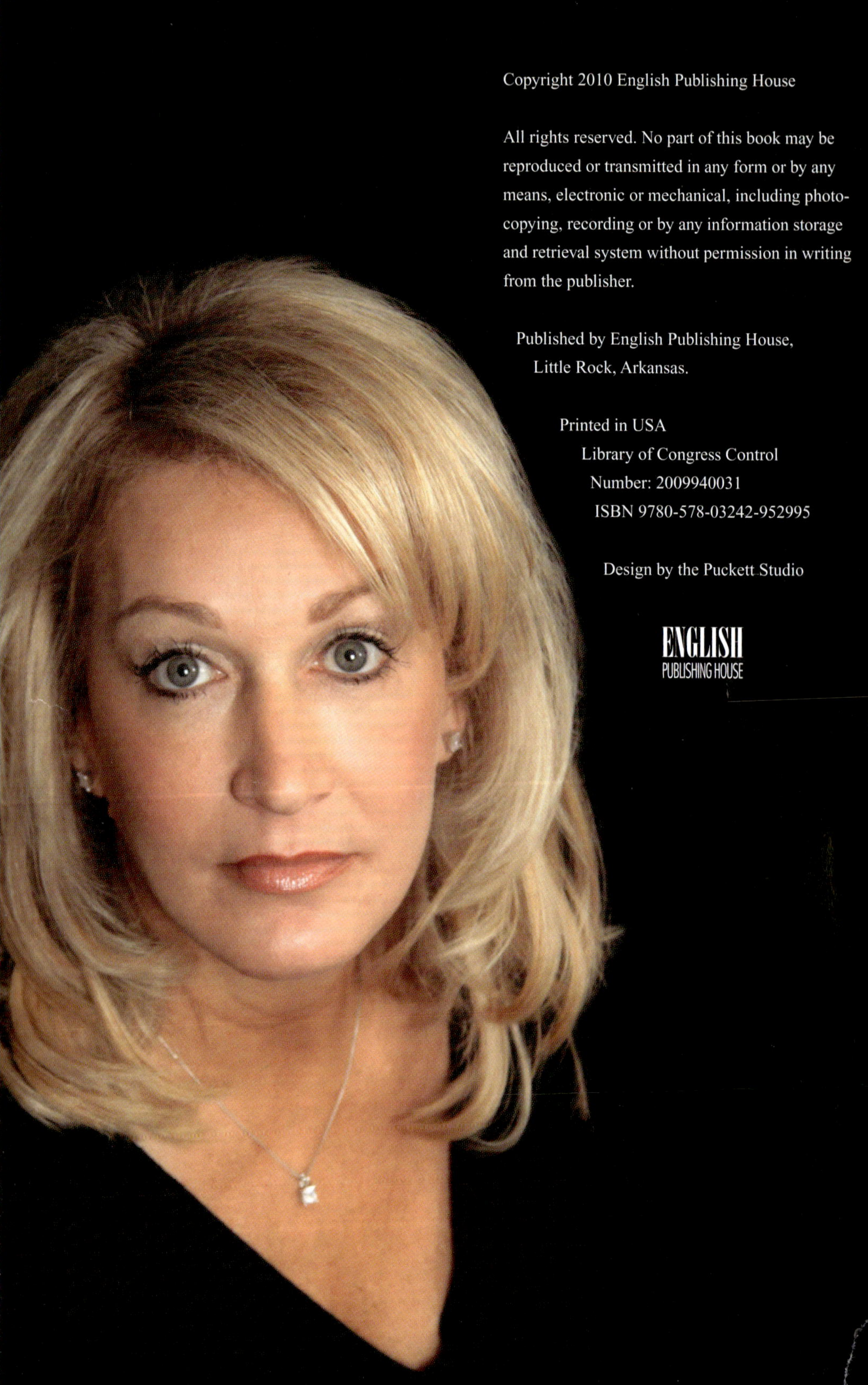

Published by English Publishing House, Little Rock, Arkansas.

Printed in USA
Library of Congress Control
Number: 2009940031
ISBN 9780-578-03242-952995

Design by the Puckett Studio

ENGLISH
PUBLISHING HOUSE

Reflections of the Heart

Stories from a Cosmetic Surgeon's Practice

By Jim English, M.D., F.A.C.S., F.I.C.S.
& Betty M. Hubbard, Ed.D., C.H.E.S.

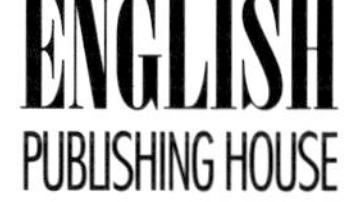

CONTENTS

ACKNOWLEDGEMENTS

We are grateful to the women who generously shared their motivations, memories
and experiences. This book would not have been possible without their
investments of time and candor.

We also appreciate the support and help of our families and friends. Their understanding
and support of this project was unequivocal, even when faced with reading numerous
drafts. They made valuable suggestions and provided encouragement as required.

The task of writing this book would have been daunting without the magnificent staff at
the English Plastic and Cosmetic Surgery Center. This family of dedicated professionals
cheerfully served as liaison between patients, physician and writer.

Though I've written several scientific articles for journals including a chapter
for a surgical textbook in facial plastic surgery, this is my first attempt to co-author an
entire book. With this professional landmark achieved, I would be remiss if I didn't take
the opportunity to give a special thanks to the one who has truly inspired me to do my
best since her birth, my daughter Chevis.

It's not easy being a physician's only child, especially mine. However, she has done
everything I could have hoped for and more. If every dad could have a daughter like
mine, they would consider themselves most blessed. She has been an inspiration to me
as I have gone about my life's work these many years. Taking care of her has
been one of the greatest rewards of my life. With heart felt appreciation,
I want to thank you for being my grown-up little girl.

P.S. I miss our time spent together. Dad

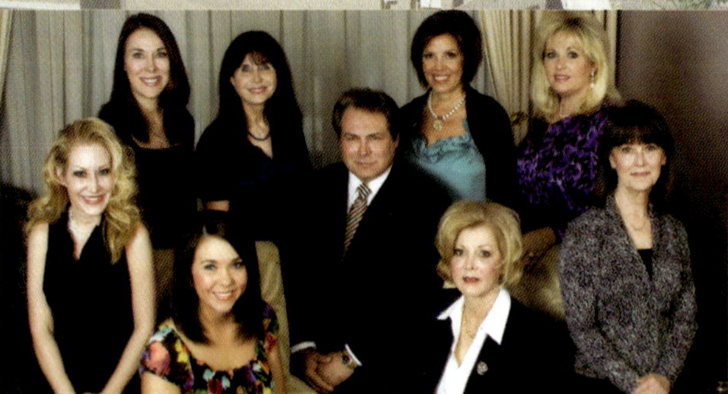

English Plastic and Cosmetic Surgery Center and Surgi-Spa Staff.

INTRODUCTION

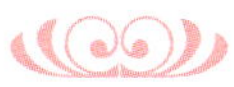

Many pamphlets and books have been written about cosmetic surgery. Additionally, numerous internet sites are devoted to plastic and cosmetic procedures. Some of these resources provide general information. Some supply descriptions of various procedures. Still others guide the prospective patient through the process of selecting a surgeon or supply "before and after" photographs. This book is different. Its goal is to present a personal, in-depth look at the experiences of individual patients within one plastic and cosmetic surgeon's practice.

Dr. Jim English, a facial plastic and cosmetic surgeon in Little Rock, Arkansas for the past 25 years, authored the book's first chapter. In it, he provides autobiographical information, along with the insights and motivations behind his life's work.

Each of the sixteen subsequent chapters presents one woman's story of her experience with their surgery. All of the women are patients of Dr. English and collectively, represent a cross-section of his clientele. They reveal their thoughts, feelings and encounters related to cosmetic surgical experiences in face-to-face interviews conducted by Dr. Betty Hubbard, a certified health education specialist. Each story is accompanied by the doctor's comments regarding the patient and her surgical case. To protect the privacy of the women who were so forthcoming and gracious in telling their stories, we have given them fictitious names.

Some of the women have experienced only one procedure while others have undergone several. The before and after photographs illustrate the changes resulting from their procedures. Note that many of the photographs reveal not only physical but emotional changes that occurred over time.

The last part of this book contains fact sheets about facial plastic and cosmetic procedures. While this information is not exhaustive or comprehensive, it does provide the basic information about the procedures described in this book. These procedures are among the most common cosmetic surgeries that are increasingly chosen by both women and men.

It should be noted that aesthetic surgery is different from most surgeries. It is one of the few surgical experiences in which the patient takes control. The patient chooses the date, the surgeon and the procedures that are performed. The motives and expectations also distinguish these surgical procedures, for instance, a facelift from curative surgeries such as a cardiac bypass. Although differences can be ascribed to surgeries that are cosmetic, all surgeries have one goal in common, to improve the patient's quality of life. A woman who experiences a boost in her self esteem after a face lift may enjoy emotional benefits comparable to a patient who has increased stamina following bypass surgery.

Research on the benefits of aesthetic surgery shows that patients can expect an increase in self image and self confidence. These benefits have contributed to an increase in the popularity of these procedures of over 100% in the last decade. During the last year for which statistics were available*, women accounted for 80% of these types of procedures. Men made up 20%. The top five procedures for women were liposuction, eyelid surgery, breast augmentation, facelift and tummy tuck. The five procedures most requested by men were hair restoration, liposuction, eyelid surgery, male breast reduction and nose surgery.

Persons of all ages elect to have facial plastic and/or cosmetic surgery. However, as would be expected, the average age varies according to the procedure. For example, the average age of persons requesting ear enhancement surgery is 27 years. The average age of patients who have nose surgery is 32. Persons who have breast augmentation, male breast reduction and liposuction are 32 years, 35 years and 41 years respectively. The average age of those undergoing hair restoration and tummy tucks is also 41. The average age of persons who have eyelid surgery is 49. The average age of those requesting facelifts is 54.*

The average costs for the most popular cosmetic procedures range from $3984 for eyelid surgery to $7241 for a facelift. Other common surgery costs are $4243 for liposuction, $5066 for breast augmentation and $6037 for a tummy tuck. Average costs for procedures performed for males are $5868 for nose surgery, $5280 for hair restoration and $3656 for male breast reduction.*

In the vast majority of cases, this type of surgery is not covered by health insurance, however, payment plans are available to patients who wish to finance their procedures and pay for them on a monthly schedule. These plans are offered by independent providers who market their services through physicians' offices. The patient completes the required paperwork and submits it in the office. The interest rate is determined by the patient's credit history.

This introduction to Dr. English's surgical field creates a backdrop for the stories, photographs and information presented in this book. You may simply be curious about the motives and experiences of women who choose cosmetic procedures. You may be a potential patient who contemplates the pros and cons of having surgery performed now or in the future. Whatever your reason for reading this book, we trust you will gain insight and a personal perspective from the surgeon and patients.

*Statistics were gathered and prepared in February, 2008 for the American Academy of Cosmetic Surgery as part of the 2007 procedural census.

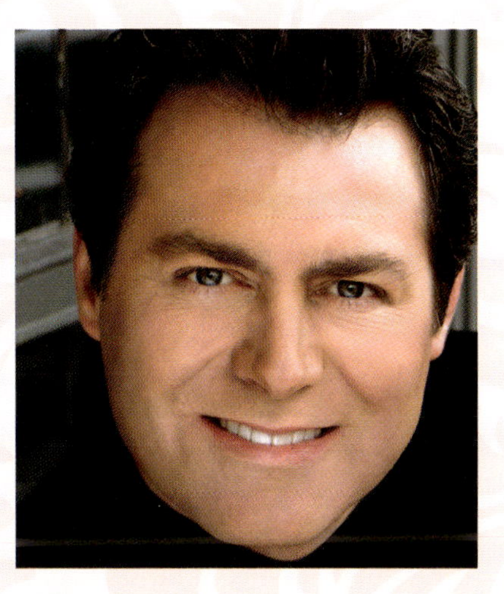

THE SURGEON'S STORY

THE SURGEON'S STORY

Stories. We all have them and their sum total makes up our collective history. Historians provide a glimpse into the expansive past with accounts akin to our own and scribes of Holy Writ provide human-interest vignettes from other perspectives. These and other texts help us better understand who we are, where we come from and what decisions we might make to avoid the mistakes of our ancestors. Though we may choose to ignore teachings from the past, the idea of a collection of stories from my surgical practice meant to inform the reader seemed reasonable. Why? Although we are each wondrously and marvelously made more similar than not, there is that inalienable right to marvel at our own individual uniqueness and think that we possess something others don't. Often over twenty five years of practice, a patient's history has led me to realize that his or her life's narrative bore an uncanny resemblance to one I had heard either recently or many years previous. Though I never tire of discussing the aesthetic design of my patients and their preoperative decisions, I've wanted my own source of written information from their past stories. In collecting those experiences, my hope is that this book might assist in answering your questions about my surgical field especially when your desires and needs reflect others that I have known.

This book as far as can be determined, is similar to none other in my field. Within its pages are the historical perspectives of my patients and their responses to the whys and wherefores that many would like to know before undergoing plastic, cosmetic and/ or reconstructive surgery. The authors hope that their surgical biographies will touch others so that when they reach for answers to similar questions, they will reflect on the responses of those recorded here.

Before we share their experiences, I shall relate my own story in hopes of giving insight into my choice of this profession and the belief system I employ in its day-to-day routine.

My siblings and I were raised in rural Arkansas. Two events consistently punctuated our existence, farm work and Sunday worship services. The former gave me a strong work ethic and the latter a sense of purpose. As youngsters, we were in the fields long before the sun reached its zenith and we gathered hundreds of pounds of produce for market daily. Reaping the harvest that day and seeing it placed in the grocery bins that afternoon was extremely satisfying. Occasionally, we would retire to the comfort of our home during the heat of the day. There we would can vegetables and quilt blankets. Early on, our mother, grandmother and great grandmother would train us in the art of sewing and fabric design. Our minds and hands were kept busy as we learned the intricacies of stitching and the spatial orientation of the pieces that fit together. Once in a while, our maternal mentors would allow us to devise the patterns and themes for the design of the quilts. At an early age, I learned about aesthetic design and it became important to my life's vocation.

Though the days spent in those endeavors were long and arduous, they allowed our family the time to become closely knit. The work provided each of us a comparative example by which to gauge future work environments and what it took to provide not only for ourselves but also for others. The opportunity of being raised in such a traditional manner with Christian core values would one day propel each of us into our respective occupations. My brother made his mark in finance before retiring to his lifelong love of automobiles and after raising three daughters, my sister became a registered nurse. She works alongside me now. My family has continued to be a wonderful bastion of support to me throughout my life. What a gift to have had such a wonderful upbringing!

Though the time spent with my family was invaluable, after eighteen years I said goodbye to that incubatorial stage and embarked on the next level of development, fourteen years in classrooms and hospitals to obtain the necessary requirements for three certifying boards required for my chosen field of surgery. Because of the excellent preparatory experience in the public school system of Arkansas, my four years of college was an extension of high school which allowed me to work while taking a full load of courses. I loved math and science and still do since I believe that our universe was created for us in such a way that we can enjoy it while learning its intellectual intricacies. With cach passing day either at work or in school, I gained an appreciation of life as a God given gift and became committed to make the best of it.

Graduating with a major in biology and a minor in chemistry after four years, I went on to medical school. Much to my chagrin, it was not an extension of college. The first week, one of my professors told our class to forget all that we had learned for they would replace it with their own body of knowledge. Lectures, reading, memorizing texts and weekly tests comprised my life for the next two years. The last two years of medical training was outside the classroom and in the hospital. This intense course of study allowed little time for anything else although I did serve as class president for three of those four years.

I enjoyed learning about all aspects of the human's unique design and function as should most of us, but before anyone considers this occupation, please know that family life, recreation and most everything else not associated with medical school usually takes a back seat. (With the new federal guidelines for length of work week, working more than eighty hours a week is less likely than before.) It seemed that with each step up the academic ladder, the required commitments became more intense. It was the memories of days spent on the farm that helped me stay the course since I nor my siblings had any intentions of returning to farm life.

Following medical school, I started four and one half years of surgical programs with the best mentors in their respective fields, Dr. James Suen, a nationally renowned surgeon in Head and Neck Cancer and Dr. Gaylon McCollough, an internationally respected surgeon in Facial Plastic and Reconstruction Surgery. Dr. Suen personified the consummate hands-on academician and helped save the lives of many a cancer victim while I was with him. His ability to detect the dreaded disease and eradicate it was remarkable. At no time during the three years spent on his service did I ever lose trust or respect for him or in him. We spent long hours at the operating room table as some of the procedures required a full day for their completion. His grasp of anatomy and the nature and actions of the cancers that we battled for the lives of his patients were uncanny.

It wasn't enough for us as resident surgeons to name the arteries, veins, nerves, muscles, bones and other structures within the confines of the head and neck area, but the normal variation as well as the abnormal ones and their percentages. We learned not to question his corrections because he was never wrong, it was his passion not to be. "One of the most profound things that you can give a patient" he often stated, "was hope" and Dr. Suen could promise that in all but the most difficult cases. His telling patients not to worry and that their needs would be met as best as humanely possible prompted me to adopt that mindset in my own practice. My creed, within its limitations, became that of my mentor's: "Don't give less than what you are capable of even if it costs you more than most are willing to pay." My parents had taught me a similar concept in a nursery rhyme: "Good, better, best—never let it rest till your good is better and your better best." I taught my daughter the same rhyme. Although my current practice does not include cancer surgery, the lessons learned from Dr. Suen and taking care of his patients during those three years were invaluable and have helped me provide the same for my patients. I hope in time, that my fellows (I now train two surgeons a year in the art of my profession) will say that I conducted myself in the same manner as Dr. Suen.

The second part of my surgical training was my tenure with Dr. McCollough. He had trained under three of the most respected surgeons of his time and he combined their teachings into a codified art of surgery. He passed that surgical gift on to me. This mentor taught me to fish as per the ancient Chinese proverb, "Give a man a fish, feed him for a day, teach a man to fish, feed him for a lifetime." I learned not only how to perform the delicate surgical techniques that would benefit the patients I have come to know over the past twenty five years, but also how to relate to a clientele that requested surgery when they were not sick. This was the first time as a surgeon that I had to wrestle with the issue of elective procedures solely for the enhancement of beauty or as others would incorrectly infer, surgery for the vain. The first time I heard Dr. McCollough's response on this issue was from a lectern where he addressed one hundred or more surgeons. In his inimitable style, he stated "We all get up, comb our hair, brush our teeth, and put on the best face that we possibly can each and every day." Though simplistic, this statement gave me a starting point to form my own feelings about the vocation that I had been called to and directed in.

During the first six months of fellowship with Dr. McCollough, I participated in more than five hundred procedures. This participation was a surgical paradise for the meticulous training needed to hone the skills I now use for my own patients. Hour after hour, five days a week, the teacher taught and the student plied him with questions. The answers not only dealt with the what and the how but also the why and the when. We discussed and re-discussed all aspects of running a practice for the surgery of beautification and aesthetic enhancement of patients. The learning curve was steep but the abundance of effort by Dr. McCollough and his staff saw me through. Today, when I banter with my fellows in the operating room, I often reflect on that time when I could discuss issues on a moment's notice and know that I was getting the correct answers.

Coming back to Arkansas to establish a practice without a classroom or mentor was daunting. I remember the first time that I performed a rhinoplasty to enhance the patient's profile. (This procedure has the dubious distinction of being the most difficult to learn.) During the procedure, I felt the need to look up from the surgery and ask, "What now?" Then I realized that privilege no longer existed. No longer was someone else responsible for a patient's outcome. I was. No excuses would suffice. No lack of effort would be acceptable. Nothing short of doing my best while another was counting on me would do. Twenty-five years later, as I reflect on the lessons and all the effort bestowed on my training, I consider myself most blessed.

The consistent nature of my patient's stories continues to amaze me. Many ascribe personal values—useful or detrimental—in their decision making. For example, I've heard many times, "God made me this way and I should accept my lot in life." I never argue, but I do politely disagree. I believe that we were created in the image of God without spot and blemish. Since God makes it possible for us to be made whole spiritually, why can't we expect to be made as whole as possible physically? If God gave mankind the ability to ease suffering here on earth, we may rightly try to correct some of the flaws in our aesthetic design.

Yet, sometimes people become obsessed by this need and shouldn't have the work done until they resolve their issues or they will likely never be satisfied with their results. However, those with realistic expectations should feel free to explore improvement of their appearance if they so desire. The pursuit is not perfection (which is a man-made goal and gets further out of reach as it is approached) but rather that of excellence and should be achievable in most instances. As you read the stories of my patients and their impressions from me about their surgical issues in the pages to follow, you may see and appreciate the mindset that influenced their and my decision making process. I trust that God will richly bless any and all who are in search of knowledge and wisdom even if it concerns my life's chosen field of endeavour and that they know that He truly loves them regardless of their future aesthetic changes.

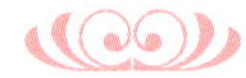

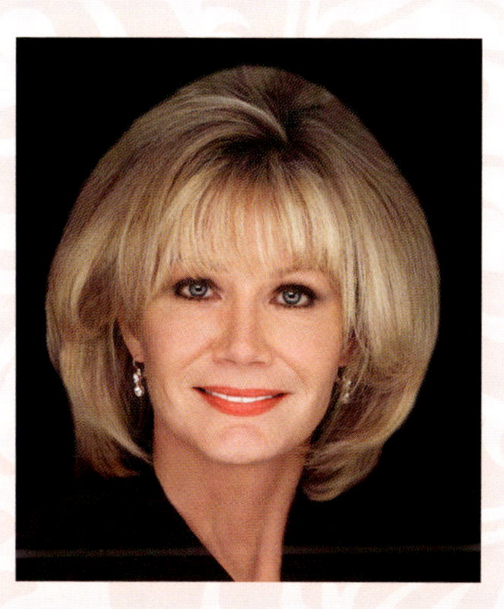

PATIENTS' STORIES

A N N A

Breast Surgery (Augmentation)

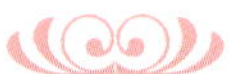

Other kids in school teased me about my small breasts. They called me, "the president of the itty, bitty, titty committee." I always felt like I never matured, like I never became a woman. When I was 13, I waited for my breasts to develop. They didn't. So I thought, "Maybe when I'm in high school." Throughout high school I kept waiting, "Maybe when I'm a senior." Even after I had kids, it didn't happen.

So on some level, I felt like a failure. This feeling began to affect my life more and more. Shopping trips were really bad. I would come home crying. Clothing just isn't made for someone who is so small. I would have to go to the little girl's section to get a bra. That was really embarrassing. It got to the point that I just couldn't handle it any more. I became depressed and had severe mood swings, especially if I needed to buy clothes.

It got harder to get ready in the morning, harder to shop, harder to do normal things. I was depressed to the point that I couldn't have a conversation because I was so self-conscious. I wore padded bras but that just made it worse because at the end of the day I had to take them off. I would look down and get depressed again.

During this time, my family was wonderful. They told me, "You're so beautiful just the way you are." My husband was especially great about trying to understand and to build my confidence. But no one could comprehend how much having small breasts upset me. I realized something had to be done. And I knew I was the one who had to take control.

I had thought about having implants for a long time, probably since I was 20 years old. But the last three years, I considered it very seriously. I searched the Internet and read a lot. I educated myself about the different types of implants and about placing implants over and under the chest muscle.

Three things bothered me about getting implants: first, the health risks. I knew complications could occur with any surgery. I guard my health very carefully. I run and like to be physically active. For example, I really enjoy manual labor like working in the yard and garden. I wanted to be sure that implants wouldn't affect my ability to stay active. Second, it bothered me that I wasn't content with the way God made me. But I believe that God knows my heart and knew I wasn't strong enough to keep dealing with the depression. Third, I was concerned about what other people would think. Subconsciously, I wanted to have the surgery then pretend that I had always had breasts. My husband helped me overcome this. He said, "You can't expect that people won't notice!"

I also thought I shouldn't spend that much on myself when I could use the money for the kids or to buy a house. But my husband gave me the surgery as a ten-year anniversary present. He asked me, "Do you want an anniversary ring or do you want a boob job?" It was a no-brainer! And it was very kind of him. I had the surgery two weeks before our anniversary to make sure that I would be recovered enough to enjoy the results.

Having the surgery has affected my life in a major way. I never knew how much my breasts bothered me until after I had the surgery. It's like throwing a rock in the water and watching the ripples moving away from the center. Every aspect of my life has been affected. I'm more open sexually with my husband now and communicate more honestly. Before, I was afraid to let people know me, to know who I am. Even with family members, I was distant before because I was always afraid of what they thought of me.

Now I can walk down the street with my head held up. I talk to people, even strangers. Before, I was uncomfortable, thinking they would notice that I had this flaw. Career wise, I feel that I can do anything that I want, where before, I had set so many limitations on myself. I would say, "Well you can't do that." I'm an artist and, even in that realm I had backed off. When you're depressed, your painting seems to be very dark and dreary. A picture I painted two weeks ago was the best one I've ever done. It was a 4x4 mural, and I completed it in one day.

My outcome exceeded my expectations. During my consultation, my doctor let me know up front that since I had so little breast tissue, they would look implanted. He said, "I'll get them as natural as I can but they are not going to look and feel real." I appreciated his honesty and I'm very pleased with how natural they look. If you saw me, you wouldn't say, "Oh, she got a boob job." You know, like you see on movie stars, where their breasts look like big balls. Mine don't look that way at all. I'm proportional.

Before surgery, my doctor measured me and pretty much chose the size of the implants to fit my hips. He said, "If you go too small, you still won't be proportional." My breastbone is very narrow so he had to special order my implants. I went from an A to a C or D, depending on the bra. I thought I might have stretch marks, but I don't. I have no visible scars, just a tiny pink mark on each breast where the incision was.

My best friend can't believe how good my breasts look. I love the shape and am so proud that I did this. I wish I had done it years ago. If anyone asked me about cosmetic surgery, I would say, "Don't wait. Do it for yourself. Don't do it for a boyfriend or your husband. It's got to work for you."

ANNA

The Surgeon's Impressions

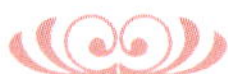

When Anna came to the office, her emotional concerns about her small breasts had haunted her since adolescence. She actually had little or no breast tissue and no fat in the breast area. There was an almost masculine morphology (structure) to her chest wall. I told her that we needed to get the implant as deep as we could so we would have as much coverage as possible. I also told her that since she had so little breast tissue, her breasts would look as if they had been implanted. This was a tradeoff that she was willing to accept because she had suffered from lack of breast development for so long.

I decided to use a high profile implant because she has a narrow chest. Chest width is important because it determines the base dimension of the implant. High profile implants on women with narrow chests tend to have a very attractive outcome with more cleavage. They also result in more anterior projection. You don't want to use high profile on someone who has a wide chest because the breasts may appear unnaturally protrusive.

Her left nipple from her sternal notch (top of the breast bone) at the neck base was 5 mm lower than the right, which is not significant. Many women naturally have that much or more asymmetry. I chose not to do anything about her asymmetry (though sometimes, if the asymmetry is a half inch to an inch, I'll do a small crescent mastopexy - breast lift - on the affected side to get the nipples horizontally matched). Augmenting a significant asymmetry will make it even more noticeable, so if the asymmetry is only a few millimeters, it's one thing; if it's a couple of centimeters (an inch), it's totally different.

Anna healed very well. Her incisions were almost imperceptible around the areolar area. She has done remarkably well from a physical standpoint in her convalescence but more importantly, from an emotional standpoint as well.

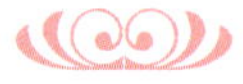

LILY

Eyelid Surgery, Forehead Lift, Facelift, Mid Facelift, Fat Transfer and Chemical Peel

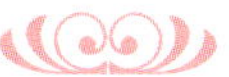

I was 54 years old and probably looked 65. My hair was gray and my teeth were discolored because I took tetracycline as a child. But I felt okay about my appearance until I had a heart attack and lost down to 70 pounds. I regained the weight but my face never filled out. Then I went through a divorce and really withdrew into a shell. During the divorce, I decided to move back to Little Rock. There I reconnected with my cousin who started making suggestions about my appearance, like coloring my hair. The change in my hair color made a difference that I liked very much. Then my cousin said, "I have this great dentist who could fix your teeth." I wasn't so sure I wanted to do that, but I got veneers and now I can't believe my smile. I was always so ashamed of my teeth.

Then my cousin began to talk to me about her friend the cosmetic surgeon. I had heard other people brag about him and knew he had a good reputation. So I made an appointment. The first time I met this doctor, I was impressed by his questions and his medical knowledge. He also cared about my overall health. He said that, because of my heart attack, I would have to get approval from my cardiologist. I also have a blood disorder and see a phlebotomist. He said my blood would have to be at a certain level before he could perform the surgery. And he wanted confirmation from both of these doctors that having surgery was okay. I also liked his rule about smoking. He said, "You can't smoke and have this surgery." I wasn't ready to have the surgery at that time because of the cost but about a year later, my cousin made the surgery possible. If I think about her kindness too much, I cry. She has just been a wonderful champion for me.

At first, I felt that I would be changing myself and wondered if I had a right to change my face. But I color my hair and wear makeup so I just didn't see much difference. Most of us want to look our best. When we do, our self-esteem goes up. We smile a little more and are friendlier. I came to understand that the surgery wasn't going to change who I was; it would just enhance the way I look. Once the cost wasn't an obstacle, I was so ready for the surgery. I wasn't the least bit apprehensive because I had a lot of faith in the doctor and everybody else in the office. The morning of my surgery, I think my cousin was more nervous than I.

I don't remember much about the surgery, just the anesthesiologist and the doctors. My next memory was at my cousin's house. She was steadying me because I was having a little trouble getting up the stairs. My head felt huge because it was bandaged. I couldn't see much because my eyes were swollen. I probably wouldn't have wanted to see myself anyway. The first four days I mostly remember being given medication and sleeping. Once I stopped taking the medication and was more awake, I called myself the bride of Frankenstein. I was very swollen. I wasn't hurting but since I had a phenol peel, I had to shower several times each day. Those stung at first. Then they began to feel so good. I told my cousin I was the cleanest guest she ever had.

When I was able to examine my face in the mirror, it was swollen but didn't have any huge bruises like I thought it would. I knew that when the swelling went down, I would look so much better. That was exciting. I went back to work two weeks after my surgery – without makeup. I was red and swollen. Everybody in the office knew about my surgery and was able to see the whole healing process. One of the girls started taking pictures once a week. Most of the women were really interested and enjoyed watching the swelling go down. They say it's been fun to see the changes. One of the very young girls recently said, "Lily, you look so good." I just loved it.

This has all been such a good experience for me. The only negative was family members who didn't approve of my surgery. My stepfather was very upset and it took me a while to figure out why. I've always looked like my mother and she died recently. He would come into a room and not even look at me. Much of the opposition from others comes from the fear that you won't look like yourself. But you can't let others' reactions wound you. It's about them. It's not about you. In the past I wouldn't have had the surgery because I want to make everybody happy. I had the surgery anyway; I decided whether they approved or not, I wasn't doing it to please them. I was doing it to feel better about myself. Now that I've had the surgery, it's made me feel even more confident because I made my own decision and followed through. The surgery has influenced every part of my life. It's been a fresh start because I feel more comfortable with myself. I had accepted that I was part of the older generation and that looking old was what my life was going to be. But mentally, I was drained by looking old. It made me feel old. Looking younger makes me feel younger.

Recently, I saw one of my mother's friends whom I hadn't seen in about 30 years. She hugged me and I said, "Do you remember me?" She said, "Of course I do!" I thought, "Well I still look like Mama – just a younger version. So I would say that a woman should have cosmetic surgery for herself – not because she wants to meet a man or so her husband won't leave. Maybe those would be good reasons for someone else, but not for me.

LILY

The Surgeon's Impressions

When I first met Lily, she looked approximately 20 years older than her stated age. She had recently experienced a divorce as well as some serious medical problems and appeared to be quite depressed. She and her cousin came to my office to explore cosmetic procedures to rejuvenate Lily's appearance. My recommendation was to begin with a dental restoration because her teeth were stained and uneven. I suggested that the dental work be followed by "the works" (brows, upper and lower eyelids, mid face and lower facelift). Later, a Baker-Gordon chemical peel would finish the rejuvenation process. Facial surgery followed by a chemical peel is like baking a cake. The surgical aspect is the cake, and the chemical peel is the icing. This type of chemical peel subtracts three to ten years from one's appearance because it tightens the skin.

Some issues must be considered when using the Baker-Gordon peel because it affects a deeper level of tissue than other peels. It causes some permanent hypo pigmentation (lightening). The skin becomes one-half to one shade lighter but the results are worth the change in pigmentation. In Lily's case, her skin was very sun damaged, having a weathered and leathery appearance and her face was heavily lined. You just can't pull out a wrinkle or crease surgically. Surgery repositions tissue that has fallen and also removes excess skin. But you can't eliminate a crease. Even if you could, it wouldn't look natural. So if a patient has lines following surgery, I follow up with a procedure to resurface the skin.

Lasers, dermabrasion and chemical peels are all resurfacing procedures. When considering chemical peels, a salon peel could be equated to a Volkswagen, a deeper peel, like a TCA peel or a Jessner peel could be considered an Oldsmobile. A phenol peel would be like a Cadillac and a Baker-Gordon peel would be the Mercedes. When I consider resurfacing or tightening lines on a face with a chemical peel, I must consider the depth of tissue that will be affected. Each of these peels creates a successively deeper wound, thus creating a better effect up to a certain point. The deeper the peel is, the more lightening of the skin and the greater the chance of scarring. The deeper the peel, the longer it takes for recovery. So I choose the particular resurfacing procedure to accomplish the patient's specific needs.

Lily had the dental restoration and facial surgery. She recovered well and has a great result. She looks much less than her stated age now and her self-confidence has sky rocketed. Her result is excellent; however, one more procedure is needed to tighten the remaining lines and wrinkles on her face. In six to twelve months I want to finish her rejuvenation process with the Baker-Gordon chemical peel.

CLAIRE

Liposuction

Last winter I got eczema on my upper thighs. That was when I realized that my belly, this big ole gut, was hanging over and onto my legs! On that day, I told my husband, "I've just got to have something done."

My husband knew this was really getting me down. When we married 20 years ago, my lifestyle completely changed. My husband didn't like to eat early. He wanted to come home, have a couple of drinks, sit around and then start cooking. We would eat dinner around 9:00 p.m.

I had been divorced for a couple of years when we married so I enjoyed cooking for him. I love to cook and, at that time, most of my meals were good country cooking. We'd have fried chicken or chicken fried steak with mashed potatoes and gravy – things that I made when my children were growing up and we were eating earlier. I didn't think much about it since I had never had a problem with weight. But over the 20 years, my whole physical being changed – my face, my body – everything.

It was hard but I finally accepted the fact that I was fat. And I also accepted the fact that I needed to make some changes to control my weight. I had always been able to do the things I set my mind to. And I was going to do this too! But, after exercising and eating more vegetables and salads for 6 to 8 months, this beat me. It was really depressing.

My body was never a problem with my husband. My body was a problem with me. When I got dressed, I would put on a latex garment that lifted me up and held me in. I always wore long shirts to disguise and hide my gut. I'm not tall so these tops made my legs look two feet long. I never wore anything form-fitting.

You can try to camouflage the way you look through your clothes and you can camouflage it in your head. You tell yourself that it's not that bad. You think you're hiding it but then you see yourself in a full-length mirror. Seeing pictures of me was really bad. I felt so self-conscious about my appearance that I stopped going out. I didn't want anybody to see me. The way I looked affected me socially and sexually. It influenced every part of my life. When my husband realized how much of a problem this was for me, he said, "You go talk to some doctors and see what they say. If they can do it, then just plan it."

The first doctor I went to see was in the town where I live. I had read articles about him in the paper so I made an appointment for a consultation. I told him, "This is not a tummy. This is a gut. Can you do something about this fat?" He looked at it and said, "Yes, I think so but it would be good if you could lose 20 or 30 pounds first. It would look a lot better." I thought, well I'd love to lose that weight. I've tried to lose it. Maybe I could enroll in one of those weight loss programs and get those 20 pounds off. So that was in the back of my mind. I talked to his scheduling nurse and saw the before and after pictures. She showed me a woman whose gut was like mine. She'd had a tummy tuck and I thought, yeah, okay, I can see the difference. So I thanked them and said, "I'll let you know." In the meantime, I knew I'd be trying to lose those 20 pounds and it would take awhile.

Two weeks later I had my appointment with the second doctor. I found myself sitting in the waiting room with many beautiful people. Nobody looked like me with my frumpy fat. I was certainly the oldest person there. Most of the people were 35 or 40 years old. They probably wanted to look more attractive for the business world. I just wanted to get the ole gut off. I thought, "Fat people don't come here." So, when the nurse took me back to the consultation room, I said, "I want to see what the doctor could do with my chin." She said, "Well, when you called you didn't say anything about your chin." I confessed that after looking at the people in the reception area, I didn't think the doctor would work with someone like me. The nurse said, "Oh, Claire, you have no idea." She told me her own story and showed me pictures.

As we talked, I began to understand that the way I felt was not unusual. Then the doctor came in and here I was in this robe. This was the part where you have to open the robe and show them what you want to change. But it didn't take long to feel comfortable – I just took a deep breath and thought, "Let 'em see it." After having children and a colonoscopy, you would think there was little left to feel self conscious about. But I wouldn't even let my husband see my gut. I was so extremely self-conscious. I hated it and didn't want my husband touching it. I laughed and told the doctor and nurse, "Ya'll have seen more of me than my husband in the last year – at least in the light!"

When the doctor examined me, he grabbed a handful of fat and said, "Okay, squeeze down like you're having a contraction." I guess he was feeling where my muscles were. He didn't talk about any surgery, strictly liposuction. I had asked the nurse, "Should I lose 20 pounds?" She said, "You'll just put yourself 6 months behind. You can get this done now and lose 20 pounds later if you want to." I thought, "Wow, what a relief." I knew if I wanted to get rid of my gut, this was the way I wanted to do it.

I don't remember much about the surgery but I do remember the next day when I came back for my follow-up appointment. I looked at myself and thought, "Oh my!" I couldn't believe there was that much change. My belly was flat! And this was strictly liposuction – no incisions. The nurse had told me, "After a few months, if you have loose skin, he can remove it." So I imagined having loose skin hanging off of me like those pictures of people who lose 300 pounds. But mine doesn't look like that. I don't think I'll need surgery. If my skin is a little loose, that won't bother me. I'm not going to wear a bikini.

But now I like myself again. And when you like yourself, you like everybody else. My husband is very pleased too. He never compliments me on anything but he'll say, "That looks good" or "That looks nice" and that's a big compliment from him. One day I told him, "You must think I'm silly because I walk by the mirror a lot." He said, "I see you doing that and I just laugh. I know you feel good and you look good too."

I didn't hide my liposuction from anyone. I told my friends I was having it done. And I couldn't wait to see them afterwards and say, "Look here girls!" If I'd known that it would make me feel this different and I'd have such a positive outlook, I would have had liposuction two years ago. A weight was lifted from me.

I would tell others that if they have something that bothers them the way my gut bothered me, "Don't wait. Don't wait another week. Make the appointments. Do what I did. Talk to a couple of doctors and see how they make you feel. Then go with whomever you feel most comfortable. I've always been a believer in getting a couple of opinions. If you're not comfortable with someone right off the bat, I don't think it's going to change. I think you have to feel that confidence. You may think that you're by yourself and it's so selfish. I felt that way at first, but I'll tell you, it's time to be selfish. Why should you live with something that bothers you so much?" I still have a big butt and big thighs but I feel good and I'm proud of the way I look. Liposuction is better than antidepressants.

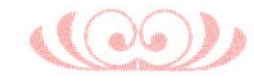

CLAIRE

The Surgeon's Impressions

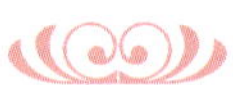

Claire is an exuberant person who enjoys life but was tired of feeling matronly. She expressed a desire for a more defined waist area. Her body type is an example of central obesity. Her arms and legs are thin, her face is a little full, but her abdominal area was inconsistent with the rest of her body. At least two steps were needed for her abdominal enhancement. The first was to reduce the volume of the anterior (front) abdomen as well as the back and flank areas. This reduction was accomplished through liposuction, which can achieve an almost circumferential gird-like reduction. Liposuction can be followed by the second step, an abdominoplasty (tummy tuck), four to six months later.

Some surgeons prefer to perform only abdominoplasty on someone who has this patient's morphology (structure). But afterward, the patient looks like a tree trunk, or worse, a girded tree trunk. If a patient truly wants a waist, significant flatness of the anterior abdomen, and as much contour and improvement as possible, the best way is to perform the liposuction first. Allow at least four to six months for the swelling to abate. Then come back and perform the tummy tuck. You'll have a much better result, much better contour and the patient will be much happier.

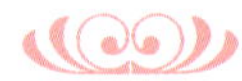

KATE

Eyelid Surgery, Forehead Lift, Liposuction, Facelift, Mid Facelift, Breast Lift and Tummy Tuck

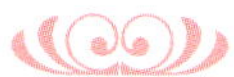

When I was 18, I married a man who had two young children, whom I raised. Three years later, I had a baby. We didn't have any money so we both worked hard and struggled for many years. We had a great marriage until the last four or five years. It was as if my husband changed when we became successful. He started saying that I was disgusting to look at. I just wasn't good enough anymore. It felt as if I had given my life to him and everyone else. My parents died within six months of each other, which was a huge shock. I thought, "Is this all there is?" Their deaths were the trigger for changing my life and I decided to make one change at a time. The first change was to get rid of my husband. So one day, he came home from work and I just wasn't there. He didn't believe that I would leave him in a million years. He's sorry now but it's too late. He killed my feelings for him.

When I left my marriage, I was 50 years-old and had sold real estate my whole working life. That business has no benefits so I had to get a job that paid well plus had benefits. That's tough when you work in sales and compete with people who are in their 20s and 30s, many right out of college. I don't have a college degree but I do have years of sales experience.

Having cosmetic surgery helped me look young enough to compete. Now I look young plus I have the experience. Most people guess that I'm in my early 40s. I've had a lot of cosmetic surgery over a three-year period. The first procedure was eyelid surgery and a brow lift because every time I looked in a mirror I saw my mother. She abused me when I was a child and I just couldn't stand seeing her eyes looking back at me. At first, my brother said I didn't need the surgery but then he saw a picture of me. He could see how much my eyes were looking like our mother's so he said, "You go have that surgery!"

The eyelid and brow lift surgeries were easy and made such a big difference in my looks that I decided to have liposuction. I love the result from that procedure because it makes such a big difference around my midsection. When you have kids and get to be a certain age, you just can't get rid of that bulge no matter what you do, so I was thrilled.

Then I had a facelift. Later I had a tummy tuck, a breast lift and a mid facelift. I've learned that there is a difference between a facelift and a mid facelift. As women get older, they get more masculine looking. Their cheeks drop and they get a wider jaw line. As men age, they have these same changes but just look more masculine. When I looked at myself, I was looking saggy and masculine. The mid facelift brought my cheeks back where they began. I always had nice cheekbones but they were hidden before.

I thought about having cosmetic surgery for about a year before my first one. During this year I did some checking on cosmetic surgeons. My good friend knew a cosmetic surgeon and spoke very highly of him. So I made an appointment. I didn't see any other doctors because I had seen a lot of "work." I was selling real estate at the time and worked with about 30 women, about twenty of whom had cosmetic surgery using a variety of doctors. One woman's hairline is too high. Another's skin is so tight that she can't smile. Another friend can't close her eyelids because they're too short. The doctor I chose wouldn't have had these results.

Two of my daughters didn't like the idea of my having cosmetic surgery. They said, "You don't need it." My youngest daughter is an RN and she was supportive from the beginning. The other two wouldn't talk to me for a month after my last surgery. In fact, they didn't spend Thanksgiving with me. One reason they reacted that way may be that there is only a 13 year difference between me and the oldest daughter. I'm 14 years older than the second daughter. Now people think that I'm their sister and that's probably hard for them. With my youngest daughter, there are so many years difference in our ages that it's not a problem. We are all on good terms now. It's been over a year now so my daughters are more accepting.

With each procedure, I've liked the result and how it made me feel. I could have never had all of these procedures at one time. It would have been just too much. Also, doing it gradually, people didn't notice the changes quite as much. They really can't tell what I've had done. They just think, "Wow, divorce really agrees with you!" Or they comment that changing my hair color has really made a difference. But the most important thing is that I look very natural. I had so much confidence in my surgeon's ability; especially after I had my eyelid procedure and brow lift. I didn't lie awake the night before surgery and I've never had any doubts about my decision. I didn't take a single pain pill even with the tummy tuck, the most difficult surgery. The discomfort lasted about three days and then I got into trouble with my doctor for doing too much.

I'm very open about the surgery I've had. I've never tried to hide it. I was showing houses the day after my first surgery even though I looked like I had been in a prize-fight. I can't think of one negative thing about having cosmetic surgery. I wouldn't hesitate to do it all again. It's helped me in my career and in my level of confidence. Cosmetic surgery has also helped me in my personal life. I just have a new spring in my step. When you marry young and stay married for 33 years, it's easy to become codependent.

I've never been vain or bought many clothes so cosmetic surgery doesn't have anything to do with how I look to other people. It is about doing something to feel better about myself. Not only did it change me on the outside, it changed me more on the inside. It's hard to explain, but it just did.

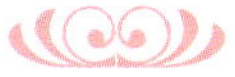

KATE

The Surgeon's Impressions

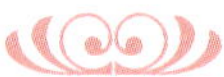

I completed this patient's facial rejuvenation in three stages. Because of Kate's job as a realtor, she could only take so much time off work to recover. When people come in and want just one procedure but need more, I accommodate their wishes even though I would like to be able to do it all at once. The more I do at one time, the better the patient's results. It would have been nice if she hadn't had to experience three separate surgeries. I can usually accomplish many procedures quickly - in two or three hours, so I don't have to worry about having someone in surgery for a long period of time.

Kate wanted only her eyes done and I thought, "If only I could do more than just her eyes." She had a lot of aging in her eye and mouth areas but not so much in the neck. There were numerous rhytids (wrinkles) around her lips and considerable sun damage. She has pretty eyes but they just didn't look happy. They looked much older than they had to. I performed a blepharoplasty (eyelid surgery) and a brow lift first. Then she came back for a facelift but I still didn't do all that I needed to at that time. Kate had some mid face descent and needed a mid facelift. She came back later for that.

I also performed body liposuction, an abdominoplasty (tummy tuck), and breast lift for her at a later time. When you look at Kate's photographs, you can see the physical changes but she was also going through a personal metamorphosis during those procedures. Now, she has completed her physical as well as her personal quest.

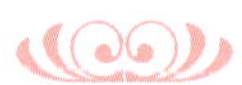

ROSALYN
Breast Surgery (Augmentation)

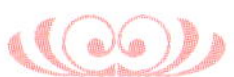

A few years ago, I never would have considered breast augmentation. I was happy with my 34B bosom after a roller-coaster ride through bra sizes ranging from A to DD. The ride began around age 12 when my breasts began to bud. My first bra was a 32B – no "training bra" for me. Due to the genetic heritage from my grandmother, my buds continued to blossom so that, by age 15, I sported a 32D chest. At 100 pounds and standing 5'2", I was a source of concern and embarrassment for my devoutly religious mother. Clothing was a challenge to find and concealing my ample breasts was paramount. By the time I went to college, I had gained a few pounds and a couple of inches but my breasts were still prominent to the point that I acquired a nickname in the dorm – R&B (Rosalyn and Boobs).

In college, I obtained a degree as well as a husband who didn't mind my rather large breasts that sometimes attracted unwanted attention. (In fact, he really liked them.) Most of the time, I could camouflage them but men would stare whenever I wore a swim suit. After a few years of marriage, I became pregnant and delivered our first child. The hormones of pregnancy and lactation worked their maternal magic and I gained another cup size. I was a 34DD until I stopped nursing the baby. Then I gradually lost some fullness and stabilized at a 34C. Another child plus another six months of nursing left me with a full B cup which seemed to fit my frame. There was no more difficulty in finding clothes that fit. I could wear almost any style shirt or dress. I felt self-confident in a swim suit or tank top during the summer months. This happy state lasted for many years – until hormones once again began playing with my anatomy. I went through menopause a bit behind schedule, at age 56. It was not a difficult transition, but as the hot flashes began to subside, so did my breasts. They began to feel like the incredible shrinking bosoms. I bought smaller and smaller bras and eventually purchased a padded bra – something that I had never done before. Well, I can tell you that there is nothing wonderful about padded bras. I felt like I had two permanent fixtures on my chest that housed the remains of my breasts - two little bottom feeders hanging out in the basement of my bra!

I decided that I could live with small breasts but the deflated versions of my mammary glands just wouldn't do. I can assure you that I tried to make peace with smaller breasts that were slowly moving south. They were certainly not an issue for my husband who liked my body "just the way it was." I researched and wrestled with my options. Option #1 was to accept the changes in my breasts and get over it. Option #2 was to have artificial devices implanted in my body. Neither option was ideal but the latter option began to have more appeal as time went on. Once I made the decision to have the surgery and my husband was supportive, I visited a cosmetic surgeon who had a good reputation. I had seen examples of his work and felt confident that he could give me a good result. The surgeon told me that I would need only breast implants and not a lift. This news was good since I hoped to avoid the additional scarring of a lift.

My hardest decisions were whether to have silicone or saline as well as determining the size of the implants. The surgeon explained the pros and cons of each type of implant. I spent hours researching silicone vs. saline. I read articles from medical journals and finally decided to go with saline. Silicone has a more natural feel, but I was concerned about the possibility of leaks. The long-term effects of silicone leaks are still unknown and there is no way to tell whether an implant has a "silent leak" except through an MRI. I have always been a very healthy person and didn't want to take the chance of the unknown. I decided that having firmer breasts was a better choice than worrying about silicone leaks.

I also spent a lot of time thinking about the size of the implants. The doctor measured my breasts and considered the size of my chest and frame before he made a recommendation. I brought my daughter when I tried on different sizes. In the end, I went with 350 cc. implants which was the size the doctor recommended.

It was déjà vu after my surgery. At first, my breasts seemed very large and my clothes were tight. I looked like I was breast feeding! But after a few weeks the swelling subsided and I went bra shopping. What a pleasure to try on a bra and fill it up. How nice to have firm and perky breasts once more. My 34C size is proportional to my frame and hips and once again, I feel self-confident in my sweaters and blouses. My husband now says that he likes everything "just the way it is." He really should go into politics!

I have to admit that I am not "open" about my breast surgery. Why? Well, I am a black woman and I don't think that the average black woman actually considers cosmetic surgery. Maybe I would be surprised if I discussed it with others, but I'm afraid that they would just think I was vain and unable to accept the aging process.

Cosmetic surgery is not right for everyone but it has been a good decision for me. It's a personal choice that should be made after much consideration. Breast enhancement is no fountain of youth or pathway to happiness. But it helps me feel more comfortable with my body, which makes me more comfortable in my life and my relationships.

ROSALYN

The Surgeon's Impressions

This patient presented to the clinic requesting breast augmentation following her childbearing years. She is a woman of average height who has a rather barrel and broad chest. Her breast mound has a wide base with relatively good volume. She has good symmetry and a small sternum (breast bone) which is preferable when trying to obtain cleavage whether the implant is placed either under or on top of the muscle. I prefer to make peri-areolar incisions because they are rather small and centrally located vs. the ones under the breast, in the belly button or in the axilla (armpit). The incisions heal nicely because they are made at the juncture of the areola and the breast skin. They tend to become almost inconspicuous over time and are not usually as visible as those placed underneath the breasts.

When discussing breast augmentation with a patient, I take many factors into account, including the patient's lifestyle. Rosalyn has grown children and young grandchildren and didn't want huge breasts. She just wanted to have the breast mass and form that she had 20 years ago. I talked with her about putting the implants under the muscle to give her the best possible breast shape and to decrease the chance of encapsulation. Encapsulation is the formation of scar tissue around the entire implant that can cause the breasts to feel hard and/or have a distorted appearance. Encapsulated breasts may also be painful. This and other post operation complications are less frequent now due to better implants, improved techniques and medicines that can usually prevent excess scar formation.

I also discussed with Rosalyn the type of implant (saline vs. silicone), the particular covering the implant shell would have (smooth vs. textured), and the shape of the implant (high profile vs. moderate profile vs. low profile). Subsequently based upon her lifestyle, her body, her request and her need for additional size, we chose a smooth shelled, moderate profile, saline implant to be placed under the muscle through a peri-areolar incision. She had the option of choosing silicone but she chose not to.

Rosalyn tolerated the procedure quite nicely. Post-operatively she developed a bit of firmness in her breasts. She didn't want to risk the chance of their becoming too firm, so I prescribed an asthma medication that has the benefit of reducing inflammation. This medication allows the breasts to soften during the first few months of the healing process. The final results for this type of patient occur, on average, three to six months following the surgery. I am pleased to report that the medication worked well and Rosalyn's results are excellent.

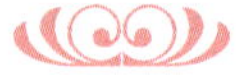

RACHEL
Buttock Implants

I've always been well-portioned and petite. But when I went through a divorce, I lost weight: from 105 pounds down to 83 pounds. The weight I lost was all from my buttocks. I tried for several years to gain it back but instead of a butt, I had loose skin. With no volume, my bottom looked flat.

Following my divorce, I had a facelift and several months later, breast implants. After that, I wanted my backside to balance out the front of my body. So I started talking to the cosmetic surgeon who had performed my previous surgeries about the best way to get a more proportional look. Initially, I had a butt lift which improved the contour of my bottom, but it didn't give me the volume I wanted. I heard about butt implants on a TV show but didn't know if my surgeon performed the procedure. When he said that he did, I didn't hesitate to say, "I'm ready!" I am very pleased with my outcome and would recommend the procedure to anyone who has lost volume and skin elasticity and also has the desire to look younger.

I'm very vain. I readily admit it. I'm going to be 29 forever. Whatever it takes to make me look younger, I'll do it! I think that any woman who has a complex about her body should get it taken care of as soon as possible. The longer you wait, the longer you suffer psychologically. You're just a happier person when you look in the mirror and feel good about yourself. You feel good on the inside as well as the outside. Don't put yourself in a financial bind, but if you can afford it, have it done as soon as you can.

None of my family members know that I've had butt implants and none of them have even noticed. Some think that I've gained weight and just look better. The only person who knows is my best friend who I've known for over 25 years. I told her that I was going to have the procedure and asked her to drive me to the clinic and take care of me afterward. I had to stay overnight in a hotel close to the clinic because I live out of town. But there really was not much for her to do. I took care of myself. As far as the recovery, I just had to sleep on my stomach for six weeks and make sure that I was careful about sanitation. After using the bathroom, I always cleaned myself with baby wipes to make sure that no bacteria spread.

Once I returned home, my friend didn't need to stay with me. She just called or came by to check on my progress. I was always comfortable and able to get around well. There was some swelling but I wasn't aware of it except that I couldn't get into my clothes. Some very nice embroidered jeans that I'd bought at a boutique were too small for several weeks after my surgery, but now I can wear them. My size has not changed. My clothes just fit much better.

I have no regrets about this surgery. It made me feel complete. I fill out my jeans and my bathing suit. Instead of looking good only from the front, I look good from all angles. I'm no longer self-conscious. A stranger actually stopped me on the street and told me I have a sweet looking butt! I can't think of any negatives about the surgery except the scarring. A person should be aware of that before having this done. My scar is a small line, shaped like a "V" along the top of my butt cheeks. The surgeon placed it in the same location as the scar from my butt lift to avoid additional scarring. It's only been four months since my surgery and I know that the scar will continue to fade over time.

I'm not open with others about my decision to have surgery. My family would be totally against it because they think I'm beautiful just the way I am. To prevent any issues, I remain secretive about it. But, if I heard someone in a store who was trying on jeans and commenting that she wished she had a bottom, I would tell her, "Hey, I didn't have one either." I would show her my results and tell her about this surgery.

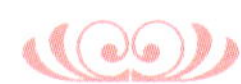

RACHEL
The Surgeon's Impressions

I first met Rachel in 2002 when she scheduled a consultation for facial rejuvenation. She is approximately 5' 4" tall and had a look of emaciation in her face because she is ectodermic. This is an embryonic term that means the individual has very little body fat. Rachel's muscles and sinew are also of a fragile nature. However, she went through a very successful facial rejuvenation and several months later, decided that she wanted larger breasts. During her breast consultation appointment, I noted that she had rather well-developed breasts that were pseudo-ptotic which means that the nipple is in a desirable position but the rest of the breast is located below it. Her breasts were deflated because of her ectodermic morphology (structure). Rachel decided that she wanted relatively large implants for her small frame. As a result of the facelift and the breast augmentation, she became a very striking woman.

Sometimes in the field of cosmetic surgery, one procedure leads to another and then another. In Rachel's case, the ten to twelve years of improvement in her face and the enlargement of her breasts drew attention to fallen and flat buttocks. Loose skin hung down over her buttock crease area. She desired improvement in this area so I discussed a buttock lift with her.

I performed the surgery by making a small but rather lengthy incision across the upper pole of the buttock in a "V" shape so that Rachel could hide the scar under a pair of French cut panties or a bathing suit. The procedure lifted the superior (upper) portion of her buttocks quite nicely and pulled much of the loose skin up above the buttock creases. However, due to her ectodermic type of morphology, Rachel still lacked buttock volume. Because of her desire for more fullness we decided to place buttock implants.

In order to prepare for the surgery, I ordered sizers to determine which implant would best fit Rachel's buttock shape. She needed volume in the lower portion of her buttock region but because she is so small in stature, the overall size and shape of the implant had to be individualized. Her upper hips were narrow but overall she had a relatively long axis (vertical length) of the hip mound. As a result, individualized implants with a special type of surface contour were made by a well-known and reputable company in Nevada. These implants were not only the exact size needed but also the size that she desired. It's crucial to place buttock implants in an appropriate plane of dissection. Because Rachel has little muscle mass and the implants needed to be placed low in the vertical axis, I decided to place them under the fascial plane (skin and connective tissue) and on top of the muscle. This placement decision is similar to the choice a surgeon has in dealing with breast implants. The surgeon must decide whether the best placement is under the muscle versus on top of the muscle versus somewhere in-between. Because Rachel had already had a buttock lift, I placed the implants through the same incisional scars.

The post operative convalescence for butt implants may be somewhat more difficult than other procedures because the patient is not able to sit or lie down on the implants for several days following the surgery. The overall physical hygiene must be exceptional to prevent any type of post operative infection.

Three months after her surgery, Rachel brought in several types of bathing suits to pose for her post operative photographs. She has gone from skin and bone six years ago to a curvaceous, voluptuous woman who feels very comfortable with her body. I am proud of the results obtained by Rachel. She made a decision after a life crisis and followed through, not only from a surgical standpoint but by incorporating a lifestyle change. She has now retired from her job of many years and is enjoying her life with a much rejuvenated face and an enhanced body profile.

Implants are not for all who are unhappy with their buttocks. In fact there is a more appropriate procedure for people who have unwanted fat in other parts of their bodies. The surgeon can suction that fat, prepare it, and then re-inject it into the buttock mound. This procedure produces a nice buttock contour. Sometimes the surgeon puts in as little as a pint in each mound but may re-inject as much as a quart and a half, depending on the desire of the patient and the amount of fat that can be suctioned. This procedure, sometimes called the "Brazilian butt lift," may be performed because some people do not have adequate adipose tissue in their buttocks to give them the volume that is now synonymous with an attractive look. However, what's attractive today may not be deemed attractive tomorrow so I am careful about making recommendations regarding buttock size and contour.

LAURA

Eyelid Surgery, Forehead Lift, Facelift, Fat Transfer and Chemical Peel

aving a facelift was a spiritual and emotional choice as well as a physical one. I believe that I have been put on this earth to be the best person I can possibly be. I believe that God wants to open the windows of heaven and pour down His blessings. He wants me to be beautiful—spiritually, emotionally and physically. The cosmetic surgeon I chose is a very spiritual person and that was a part of my decision. I saw the surgeon as God's tool or conduit. I placed my trust in God and took action.

After the surgery, my life changed tremendously. I was never overweight, but I certainly wasn't in good shape. I started working out and taking better care of myself in other ways. I know now that I'm worth it. I got a new hair cut, new makeup and new clothes that I could afford. And I noticed many changes in small things, like taking the trouble to contact somebody to work out with and having guys hold the door for me. These were new behaviors for me. Another change is the way people relate to me. It's remarkable the number of men who come up and say, "I really like your hair cut." Or, "You've lost weight haven't you?" They know that something about me is different; they just aren't sure what it is. Sometimes I go into a store and see someone I've known for years. They say, "Oh Laurie, you look fantastic."

I started a new job which I love. I work with kids in a clinic. Few older people work with pediatric patients and I have no doubt that cosmetic surgery benefited my career. I've been working as a speech pathologist for over 30 years. I enjoy what I do and I want to continue; looking younger makes a person, particularly a woman, more marketable.

I considered having cosmetic surgery for at least five years. During this time, I looked for women who had facial cosmetic surgery. I wanted to talk to them about their doctors and whether or not they were satisfied with their results. Finding women who were willing to admit to having this kind of surgery was a challenge: however, I did find them and learned there were two doctors that everyone seemed very pleased with. I consulted these two doctors, and learned that they had different opinions and recommendations.

The first doctor I interviewed wanted to do something with the muscles in my neck. As a speech pathologist, I know that any muscular change can make a difference. So I was concerned about that. The second doctor didn't mention doing anything with the muscles, plus I was more sold on what he proposed. I thought I would have several procedures at different times. But he gave a rationale for doing everything at once. If I just took care of the jowly part of my face, then my forehead would look older. He also talked about my eyes and the surface of my skin. Overall, I was convinced that he knew what he was doing. This doctor seemed to be looking at my whole face and that helped me make the choice between the two surgeons. Also, I had a comfort level with him. I was looking for a perfectionist and would recommend that anyone who is looking for a cosmetic surgeon do the same—look for a person who pays attention to the details.

Besides finding a doctor, I also had to get someone to take care of me. I didn't want my elderly mom to try to care for me so I recruited my best friend. She was available at the time I wanted to have my surgery so I stayed at her place where I didn't have to climb stairs. She took charge of my medicine because I was out of it and because I have hesitations about taking pain pills. There is a family history of addiction so I wanted my friend to supervise that part of my recovery. It's very important to have someone to take care of you for the first 48 hours.

After a couple of days, I moved over to my mom's and stayed there for another 12 days. Overall, my recovery was pretty uneventful. The cosmetic surgeon and his staff were available any time I had a concern. It was clear that they were all experts in their area and that they all cared about me. Once, a psychiatrist who is a friend of mine told me, "I've never been sued for malpractice and I think it's because I care. If patients know you care, they will never sue you." I think he's right.

Now, my friend wants to have a facelift. She says, "That must have really hurt, but on the other hand, you look great!" Several months ago, my mother put out my high school picture saying, "You look like yourself again." Before I had the surgery, I felt that I didn't look like myself any more. It was like I was becoming invisible. I don't feel that way at all now because of the changes in my appearance and my relationships. But the relationship that is most affected by my surgery is the one with myself. I have less money in my bank account now but I can't think of any investment that has paid off as well. I don't have a man in my life and that's not to say that I wouldn't have one. But now, the primary person I'm working on is me. If I find a man who's good enough for me, then I'll see. . . .

LAURA

The Surgeon's Impressions

Laura was very frank, indicating that she had already consulted two or three other surgeons. As we discussed her case, I outlined the procedures recommended for her facial rejuvenation: brow lift, upper eyelids, and a facelift with some fat in the marionette lines (lines extending from the nose toward the mouth) and middle cheek area in conjunction with some skin resurfacing around her mouth and lower eyelid region. Subsequently, Laura called to schedule the recommended procedures. She recovered well following the surgery and, each time she came for follow-up, was more pleased with the results than the time before.

The photographs of this patient indicate marked improvement in her chronological appearance. One feature that contributes to this improvement is her anterior (front) neck skin: It has a less "crepey" appearance. In addition, her marionettes are not as deep. Prior to her surgery, I knew that the facelift and the brow lift would not address the gauntness in her mid-face area. I like to lift that area if there is enough tissue. Rejuvenating a face involves not only relocating tissue to a more youthful position and tightening loose skin, but also filling in a face that's gaunt. Some people lose facial volume as they age while others gain facial volume. This patient had lost some facial fat in her cheek area and the remaining fat had descended. Her face is somewhat angular which is easier to rejuvenate. If the patient has good bony projection of her cheeks and chin, re-draping the soft tissues produces a more dramatic result with less trauma. In Laura's case, I took abdominal fat, centrifuged it and placed it in her mid-face to create a more pronounced cheek area. That's what stands out to me as being the most remarkable part of her rejuvenation process. The rejuvenated mid-face gives her a more youthful appearance.

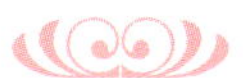

EMMA
Skin Cancer Repair

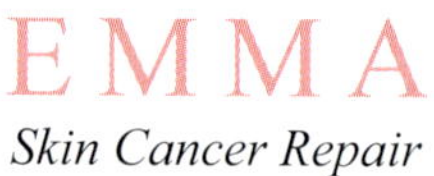

I had a little red spot under my right eye. It was not raised. It didn't itch and it didn't hurt. But I knew that I needed to have it checked so I made an appointment with a doctor in my town. This doctor wasn't able to diagnose the spot and advised me to come back in six months. I just didn't have a good feeling about my experience with him, so I went to a dermatologist in a nearby city.

He wasn't able to diagnose the spot either but froze it off. This freezing didn't seem to have any effect, so I waited about six more months and made another appointment with him. He told me he wanted to try freezing it again, which he did, but he made me promise to come back for a follow-up visit. The spot seemed to get better for a while but it didn't completely disappear.

Six months to a year later, I had my follow-up appointment. At this time, the dermatologist decided to perform a biopsy. In all, these doctors' visits and waiting between appointments spanned five to seven years. When the biopsy results came back, the diagnosis was basal cell carcinoma. I had cancer!

After the diagnosis, the dermatologist told me a plastic surgeon from his group would meet with us. The plastic surgeon examined me and then the doctors went out of the room to talk. My doctor came back and said, "The plastic surgeon says he doesn't do this sort of surgery." I knew that this surgeon did all of the reconstruction for the dermatologists in this group! Something was very wrong. I felt he didn't want to operate on my face, for whatever reason. Then the dermatologist referred me to a doctor who does nothing but reconstructive surgery around the eyes.

This doctor said, "During the surgery, I'll cut a circle around your cancer to be sure I get all of it. It's likely that I'll have to take some skin from one or both of your eyelids to graft under your eye. You'll need to wear a patch over your eye for a short time. Eight to ten months after the surgery, you'll be able to cover the scar with makeup." I scheduled the surgery with this doctor but, once again, I just didn't have a good feeling. So I went to another dermatologist who specializes in cancer surgeries. My daughter had been to see him and knew that he performed a procedure called "Mohs surgery."

In this surgery, the skin cancer and any "roots" that may have grown out from it are removed. This procedure has the best cure rate but the surgeon doesn't know in advance how much tissue will need to be removed. I would have to go into surgery not knowing how bad the cancer was or how much of my facial skin would be removed. This uncertainty plus another incident created a lot of anxiety for me.

I worked with a woman who had terrible scars on her face. She looked mangled. I assumed she had been in a horrible car accident. Then I learned that the scars were from skin cancer treatment. I learned about this after my diagnosis and before my surgery, so I was very upset. She had a procedure called a "flap" where skin is removed from another area to cover the place where the skin cancer was removed. I became so anxious that every day, I would cry all the way home—an hour's trip—because I didn't know how I could face going from looking normal one day to looking deformed the next. How could I willingly let someone cut on my face?

I rode to an out-of-town conference with a woman from my company and told her about my situation. She told a friend who called me and said, "I wish you would go see my doctor. He's a cosmetic surgeon and he does a wonderful job." She had a skin cancer removed and a mini-facelift at the same time.

So I called this doctor's office and told his nurse that I really needed an appointment. I said, "I'm just so upset about this, can I come in?" I was so desperate. At my appointment, this doctor showed me pictures of work he had done. He was not overconfident and I liked that. I immediately felt comfortable in his office and knew he was the one to perform my reconstructive surgery. But I was still anxious. I told him, "I can cover this spot with makeup. What will happen if I don't have this surgery?" He said, "It will spread."

He told me about a man who had a cancer on his right cheek and wouldn't let anyone remove it. When the cancer got large, he grew a beard to hide it. Eventually, the cancer spread to his right eye and blinded him before it spread to his brain. The man was in his 40s. There is a reason why the sign for cancer is a crab. It keeps growing and spreading out from the site. The doctor also said that he might have to do a flap if a large area of skin was removed. But that he would do everything possible to avoid that. I began praying that I would be able to accept having the surgery.

The day before my surgery, I was talking to a woman at work. I had not told her about my cancer. She had a new grandson who was having seizures constantly. She was also dealing with serious alcohol problems in her family. I thought, I'm stressing about the way I'm going to look? I have a happy marriage and a healthy family. If I have scars, so be it! A sense of peace came over me. I knew I would get through whatever happened.

The dermatologist began removing my cancer at 9:00 a.m. After it was removed, there was just a big, gaping hole in my face—about the size of a silver dollar. Then I went to the cosmetic surgeon's office for the reconstruction. All of this was done with a local anesthesia, so I was awake the whole time. I'll never forget lying on that gurney and seeing the doctor sitting in the corner with his head in his hands. He was probably praying. I thought, how horrible to put this responsibility on this man. I said,

"I see you sitting over there worrying and I know that you will do the very best job that you can. So don't worry about it."

When I looked at my face immediately after the reconstruction surgery, it didn't look like a scar. It looked more like a slit- one that was perfectly knit together. I wore special brown tape for six months and, at one point, my eye began drooping because the scar was pulling it down. I hadn't noticed it but my doctor caught it right away. He is a perfectionist and knew how to maximize my healing. He and his staff treated me like the most important person in the world, calling me every day for two weeks to see how I was doing.

At a follow-up visit, an intern came in to see me. He said, "I've seen your pictures and I can tell you that your doctor performed a miracle. With some procedures, you can go in later and tweak the work. But for a situation like yours you have one shot to get it perfect." I think that's exactly what my doctor did. If I hadn't had such a good result, I may not have wanted to be with the public – and I have a very public job. I may have become more reclusive. In my case, reconstructive surgery made the difference between looking normal and being disfigured. There is no value you can put on that.

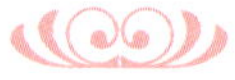

EMMA

The Surgeon's Impressions

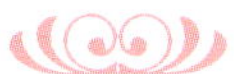

When I met Emma, she was fearful and dealing with uncertainty. She had been telling doctors about the lesion under her right eye for quite some time and it had not been managed adequately. The lesion was a morphea-form basal cell carcinoma, a type of skin cancer. There are two basic types of basal cell carcinoma. One is a nodular form that grows like a wart. This type can be easily identified and is easier to cure. The other type is insidious and grows like Bermuda grass in a garden. "Cancer" means "crab" and that's a good description of how this type of cancer grows, sending tentacle-like projections throughout the tissues. If you leave those projections when you take out the primary lesion, you'll have recurrent cancers springing up in different areas.

Emma had seen an excellent Mohs surgeon (a dermatologist specially trained in an advanced treatment procedure for skin cancer) here in town. He diagnosed the cancer and explained that it was close to her eyelid. He told her that her situation was not good, especially since she'd had the lesion for quite some time. This surgeon explained that, when the cancer was removed, she would lose a substantial part of her eyelid and possibly its function. She had also consulted an oculoplastic ophthal-mologist (doctor who specializes in eyelid surgery) who was an excellent surgeon. He discussed the possibility of using a skin graft for reconstruction following the removal of the cancer. Emma wanted a second opinion.

At her first appointment, Emma questioned my being able to do the reconstruction. I explained that one of my specialties included head/neck cancer and its repair and reconstruction. I told her that I would want to avoid using a skin graft. In my opinion, using a skin graft to reconstruct that area of her face would not give her the best result. I don't like skin grafts because they always look like skin grafts. Whenever possible, I use normal tissue from an adjacent area. That's the best way to reconstruct this type of defect. I explained that, instead of using a skin graft, I would make ex-tended incisions on her face and then move soft tissue into the defect. The extended incisions would enable me to not only repair the wound but to provide support to the lower eyelid. The tendency in eyelid reconstruction surgery is for the lower lid to pull down and show too much of the sclera (the white of the eye). That creates a stark and abnormal appearance.

Following the removal of her cancer, Emma had the tissue loss that was predicted. But, until she saw it, she could not appreciate the effect this loss would have on her appearance. Then as delicately as possible, even though she was scared to death, I talked with her about the repair. She basically said, "Just do the best you can and I'll do what I have to do to accept the results of the surgery."

I made one incision from the wound down along the right side of her nose, toward her upper lip. The other incision extended from the wound under her right eye toward the right ear. I didn't waste any tissue so it could cover the wound and slide up under the eyelid to provide support. Her surgery and recovery went very well. Her results attest to that. Emma has no recurrent disease after 24 months so her odds of cure exceed 98%. She looks phenomenal and is very happy with her result. So am I.

A graft would have looked indented and not matched the rest of the skin in that area. The pigmentation would have been different as well. However, the oculoplastic ophthalmologist is an excellent surgeon. I would let him operate on me. It just goes to show you that two different surgeons may have two different ideas about how to reconstruct a defect.

SARAH

Facelift and Chin Implant

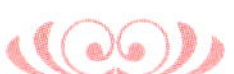

I have a childhood memory from when I was about six years old. I'm standing in the living room of my grandfather's house looking up at the wattle under his chin. I think, "I'm never going to have one of those."

But two or three years ago, I started noticing that I was getting my grandfather's wattle. I just couldn't stand it. I wasn't bothered by any of the other changes associated with aging; my grandmother's liver spots on my hands, the blotches on my face, even my sagging jaw line. But that wattle drove me crazy.

I couldn't believe that I was thinking about it so much. I never thought of myself as someone who cared about how I looked. One day, I was complaining about my wattle at work and a co-worker said, "You should have watched Oprah. She had a program about a skin treatment that stimulates collagen. Maybe that would do something about your wattle." So after some online investigation, I made an appointment with a cosmetic surgeon who offered the skin treatment. She told me it wouldn't do much for my problem. So I said, "Thank you very much," and that I would think about my alternatives, surgical and otherwise.

I am a physician who is going to work until I drop and I'm already the oldest person in my office. I decided that, if I didn't want a wattle, I deserved to not have one. At that point, I started doing research on cosmetic surgeons.

I read about each doctor and talked to people who knew them. I looked at their Websites and read their advertisements to determine what they were actually saying. I also considered their training because I wanted someone well versed in the anatomy of the head and neck. I preferred an otolaryngologist, not just a cosmetic surgeon. I also looked at each doctor's experience, training and age. Meanwhile, I studied the various kinds and methods of facelifts and decided that I didn't want a thread lift. I narrowed my search to three cosmetic surgeons and interviewed each before making my final decision.

I chose my doctor based on several factors. His bedside manner was excellent. Also, when I came for my consultation he said, "Okay, turn sideways and clench your teeth." Then he commented, "You have a deficient chin and need a chin implant." That was practically the first thing he said to me! For 60 years I lived with my chin and never thought about it being deficient! But I went home and considered what he'd said. I thought he's right. I just thought that I had a big nose. But now I know that I had a very small chin and it made my nose look out of proportion. This doctor was the only one who said anything about my chin. I wondered why none of the other doctors noticed.

I also liked that this doctor's office was next to the hospital. That was one of the main reasons I rejected one of the other cosmetic surgeons. He does the surgery in his office and it's a long way from the hospital. I know how long it takes for an ambulance to arrive. If I'm not breathing, it's not just five minutes without air; we're talking twenty minutes to get to the hospital.

Also, I would tell anyone who is trying to decide about a cosmetic surgeon to talk to nurses. They know. One of the main reasons I didn't consider another cosmetic surgeon in town was because I talked to his former nurse. She said, "This doctor does things by the seat of his pants." This nurse had found another job because she felt uncomfortable. I didn't like that one bit.

So, I chose my doctor carefully and was ready for my facelift and chin implant. (Yes, I did have a chin implant and I really like it!) The morning of the surgery, I was in my gown and had my hair all pulled up with fifteen minutes to go until time for my surgery. The nurse said something about general anesthesia. And I said, "You're not going to use IV sedation?" She said, "No." I was very afraid of general anesthesia, I think because of my medical training. My first patient when I went into my specialty area was a woman who stroked out as a result of anesthesia.

I give the doctor and staff credit for what happened next. It was the nicest thing. The nurse, the anesthetist and the doctor all came in and sat down to discuss why they preferred general anesthesia. The anesthetist said, "You know, there is one thing to consider. If anything goes wrong, I won't have an open airway." I thought he's jolly well right! He would have to intubate me if something went wrong and that takes time. So that was it. Decision made.

I was a little wobbly for about 5 days after the surgery. Nothing hurt and I had very little bruising. I really liked the follow-up care after the surgery. Someone from the office called me every evening and that was reassuring. I'd had a poor surgical experience prior to my facelift. It was an emergency surgery and afterwards, the hospital staff got me out of bed at midnight because my insurance wouldn't pay for another night's stay. I went home along a bumpy road screaming. When I got home, I couldn't urinate. That's the kind of complication that can occur and I was too out of it to think clearly about what to do. So it was reassuring to have someone call me and listen to me complain.

I went back to work after three weeks even though I probably needed only two. I had a lot of accumulated leave so I took it. Before I left work I told everybody what I was having done. When I moved to Arkansas, I found out that there are no secrets here. Everyone knows everybody else. So I thought – just tell. However, I didn't tell my family until after the surgery. I had mentioned it to them when I first started thinking about it and they all said, "You don't want to do that. That's ridiculous." So I thought I don't live near you so I don't have to tell you. When I finally told my family, my mother never said anything to me, but I thought she disapproved. So we don't talk about it. I don't bring it up and she doesn't either but that's how we handle most of our problems. My sister seems to be fascinated. Her husband said, "Well I suppose you'll want that next."

I still have some changes in sensation, like the tightness in the skin on my neck but it doesn't bother me in the least. I just didn't expect it. I don't have that windswept look that you see in some people who have facelifts. In fact, I don't look a lot younger. I really didn't want that. I just feel better. I don't look in the mirror and pull the skin on my face back any more. Sometimes, I'm surprised that I actually did it. My facelift was not a huge thing, not a sexual thing, not a matter of young or old. I don't mind looking older. I just didn't want to have that wattle.

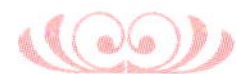

SARAH

The Surgeon's Impressions

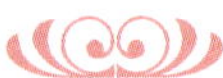

This patient is a physician who wanted her face to reflect a professional appearance as well as her vibrant lifestyle. She had some facial morphology (structure) that needed to be dealt with to help her achieve the look she desired. Most significantly, she was unaware of her weak chin. She knew that she had a significant submental wattle (sagging skin beneath the chin) and loose skin around the jaw line. But it was the lack of an adequate chin that really exacerbated the aging in her lower face and neck. So I discussed that with her. She seemed surprised at my assessment but, post surgically, she appeared to like the change in her chin as much as the results of her facelift.

Sarah also had thick skin. This type of skin is somewhat unusual for a woman. Thicker skin is good because it doesn't stretch back as much as it would if it were thin. The down side is that it's harder to remove an adequate amount because it's not as elastic. In a facelift, I may take out one to two inches of skin on each side. For someone with thick skin, you can't get that much out because it won't stretch as much. Also, she had more of a rounded face. People who have round faces tend to not have as good a result. It's easier to achieve a more dramatic outcome with someone who has an angular face.

Placing the chin implant improved her angularity. Her cheekbones were adequate and the chin really helped significantly change her face to achieve an attractive appearance.

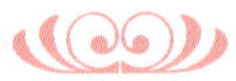

SOPHIE
Facial Reconstruction

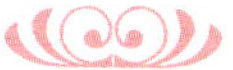

My world changed on July 29, 1992. I was in an automobile accident that caused serious internal injuries and crushed most of my face. I have no memory of the car crash itself but remember that it happened on a Wednesday night. I was on my way to church to sing in the youth choir. We lived on an old and very narrow country road. I was driving my small car. My mother wanted me to take her car which was larger but it had fresh vegetables in it so I took mine. Another driver crossed over to my side of the road and my car wrapped around a tree. The crash happened not 300 yards from my house. My mother heard it and was at the crash site within a few minutes. I kept telling her that my leg hurt and that it was hard to breathe. I also complained about my head. Blood was spurting but I could still see even though my eye socket was broken. When the swelling began, I saw double. It took almost an hour for the paramedics to get me out of the car. My cheekbones and nose were crushed. My forehead was concaved one inch, making my chin look very abnormal as well. The paramedics didn't know if I would be able to keep my legs because of their position in the car.

I was rushed to the hospital where a plastic surgeon happened to walk through the emergency room. I had 60 fractures in my skull. The doctor on call had my head wrapped and it would not allow my brain to swell. The plastic surgeon said, "No, this is not appropriate. We need to allow her room to swell." So he cut all of the bandaging off. My parents were not in the room at the time but my aunt was with me. She knew the plastic surgeon because they had their first job together at a local mercantile store during high school. My aunt signed him on to work on my case.

After my condition stabilized, I had to undergo major surgeries to repair injuries to my brain, chest, legs and face. The first surgery was brain surgery on August 5th. My plastic surgeon was in the operating room during the surgery and planned to take some fat from other parts of my body to fill in my forehead. But I didn't have enough fat because I was very thin at the time. So he used wire mesh to bring my forehead out.

My accident happened the summer before my senior year of high school. The brain surgeon didn't want me to start school and neither did the principal. But this was my senior year and I didn't want to be held back from my friends. I was bald when school started but I have a very strong self-image. It didn't bother me that I had no hair. My brain surgeon had to write a letter to my principal for me to wear hats. Back then wearing hats was forbidden. So I got all of these bedazzling hats that matched my outfits. For six weeks, I went to the first three periods and was home schooled for the last three periods. The hardest thing about going back to school was remembering how to study. It took me about three months and then it just clicked. I should have had more impairment than I did because between one-fourth and one-third of my frontal lobe is gone. Because of the tissue loss, I have cysts in my brain. Because at the time of the accident, a clot formed in my carotid artery I have no blood flow on the left side of my brain. However, my right side completely compensated.

In November, the plastic surgeon began the first of several surgeries that were performed over the next nine months. He used cheekbone implants because my bones were shattered. He reconstructed my nose using donor cartilage. I still have two scars between my eyes. The one on the right had a bone fragment; the one on my left is where part of the car penetrated my brow. The plastic surgeon brought those areas up so, in a future surgery, he could debride them. After the surgery, my whole face was taped and bandaged. I had a splint on my nose and gauze coming out of it. The only visible part of my face that was not yellow was the tip of my nose.

I had that surgery on Wednesday before Thanksgiving break and the next Tuesday, I went to my third period class. It was my hardest class and perfect attendance earned exemption from the semester exam. I had lost 10 pounds since the accident so I was just a stick person with a bandaged head on crutches. My teacher said, "Sophie, why are you back in class?" I said, "I'm not taking your semester test." I told her, Mother's waiting outside because I have a doctor's appointment after this period. She said, "You made your appointment for after this class?" I said, "Yes, I am not taking your test." I couldn't eat solid food for 10 days but I wasn't taking that test.

We always put our Christmas tree up after Thanksgiving; I remember lying on the couch and watching. I was fine with that because I knew my situation was temporary. What bothered me most was losing my independence. I wanted it back so badly. I was a senior and I was going through all of these surgeries. My mom had to fill my plate, cut up my meat and bring it to me. At 16 years old, the world is going to be yours and it was taken from me. But I knew it was short term. I had to look at it that way.

My appearance after the facial reconstruction is very similar to what it was before the car crash. The plastic surgeon referred to pictures that my family brought for him. The only difference to people who knew me before the accident is my nose. It was a little wider and longer before, but not by much. The plastic surgeon didn't have much of my nose left to work with. I had a dream the night before the splint and all of the bandages were removed. In the dream, everything on my face was pretty except my nose which was all crooked and horrible. And it was going to have to be done all over again. So when the doctor took all the bandages off, he handed me a mirror and said, "Did your dream come true?" I said, "No."

I am a respiratory therapist and work in home care now. The people I treat tell me that I'm a beautiful person all of the time. I always thank them for the compliment, realizing that the accident allows me to relate to them. I've been in their shoes so I tell them they have to look within themselves and find what they need to get better. My recovery gave me the ability to talk to my patients about regaining their self-esteem. I'm very open with them about my experience and the reconstructive surgery. I had to have a procedure recently and the doctor couldn't believe my medical history. What part of your face was rebuilt, he asked. When I told him, he said, "I would never have believed it."

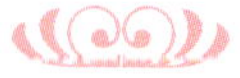

SOPHIE

The Surgeon's Impressions

I met Sophie and her family following a minor car accident that caused major trauma to her face. The patient was on her way to church when she hit a tree; she was going 35 miles per hour. Her forehead struck the steering wheel or the dashboard. She was in intensive care when I became involved in her case. Her family requested me because I had worked with her aunt during high school at a local five and dime store.

When I first saw Sophie, she had a fracture line just above the brow bone and her forehead was shoved back approximately one inch. She had fractures to her sinuses, fractures to the bones around her eyes, and fractures to her nose as well as soft tissue lacerations and damage. Her face was swollen beyond recognition, so much so that she couldn't open her eyes. She was black and blue and disoriented due to her brain injury.

Her family told me that she competed in state beauty pageants and needed to be back in the flow of things as soon as possible. So I discussed the scope of work necessary for Sophie's reconstruction with them. I developed a rapport with the family and later, with Sophie since the first few days, she wasn't able to listen to or carry on a conversation.

The initial reconstructive operation involved an oculoplastic ophthalmologist (a surgeon who specializes in eye reconstruction), a neurosurgeon and me as the facial plastic and reconstructive surgeon. After I opened Sophie's scalp with an incision that ran from ear to ear we three surgeons went to work. Two large burr holes were drilled into her skull so that a large plate of bone could be removed to expose her brain. In addition to her brain injury, Sophie also had communication from the right frontal lobe of the brain into the right eye socket. Every time her heart beat, the blood flow to the brain would communicate through the bony defect created by the accident and cause the eyeball to pulse. This is not a fatal problem but a disconcerting one when you are talking to a young woman and her eyeball pulses with each heartbeat. So we had to consider how her injuries and their repair affected both her brain and her eyes. This defect also produced a spinal fluid leak. Both were repaired during surgery.

After completing their surgeries, the neurosurgeon and oculoplastic ophthalmologist left the operating room. I was left to reconstruct the large plate of bone that had been removed from the patient's forehead and eye region in addition to the rest of her face. I pulled her forehead soft tissue back down to the level of the brow bone and fixed the bone plate back in place. I repaired the frontal sinuses and reconstructed her nose. I also fixed her broken cheeks and repaired all of her lacerations. In addition, I placed a chin implant to enhance her recessed chin profile. That wasn't part of the reconstructive surgery but it was good that she got something out of the accident other than just repair of a broken face.

The large burr holes usually are not reconstructed and the soft tissue sinks into them over time. They look like large craters the size of a small robin's egg or a golf ball. Since I knew Sophie wanted to compete in pageants, I placed a large piece of material that looks like screen wire across the entire forehead bone underneath her scalp and forehead skin so that she wouldn't have these soft tissue indentations.

Sophie recovered well and went home shortly thereafter. It is my understanding that she participated in a pageant following her surgical procedures and placed second or third. She has healed well since the initial procedure and has required only minor revision work since then. She is a beautiful young woman who is as pretty on the inside as she is on the outside.

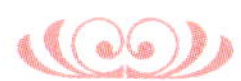

ELIZABETH
Nose Surgery

I always felt attractive even though I had a somewhat "hook nose." I disliked this feature but didn't consider changing it until my job allowed me to watch some cosmetic surgeries. I began to explore my options. Once I realized the costs and benefits of nose surgery, the decision didn't take long.

Initially, I was concerned about the risks and worried about a bad outcome. I concluded that not surviving the surgery was very unlikely. I knew that a healthy patient in the hands of a qualified surgeon has a low risk. I felt the possibility of a bad outcome was also unlikely because I would choose a qualified surgeon. I knew that if my result were less than optimal, there would be good follow up options.

I based these conclusions on reading articles and learning about the certifications for cosmetic surgeons. I talked to many who had plastic surgery. Also, as the vice-president of a surgical equipment company, I watched surgeries. I knew to consider the surgeon's training, experience, and demeanor.

The surgeon's training was extremely important to me because nasal surgery is one of the most difficult procedures. The goal is a nice looking nose that still functions well. Since my surgeon's training began in ear, nose, and throat surgery, I knew he was qualified. He also completed a fellowship with a nationally respected facial surgeon.

Good training is critical but so is experience. Each patient is different so every procedure has some variation. Years of experience add up to a confident surgeon who can make the decisions necessary during a procedure.

I also considered the surgeon's attitude. I knew the surgeon's conduct could affect a patient's result. I wanted a patient doctor. An impatient doctor may get frustrated and end a procedure before he has achieved the best result. A doctor who loses his temper in the operating room can affect the ability of his staff to perform. I had seen my doctor in surgery. He was quiet and calm and maintained a pleasant working relationship with his staff. He also strove for excellence; another quality I considered a necessity.

The thing I liked most about my nose surgery was how it improved my self-esteem. It still does 18 years later. I feel better when I see myself in the mirror or when I see pictures of myself. I feel better when I see old pictures of me and know that the feature I disliked so much has been changed. Since my nose surgery, I used the same surgeon to perform several facial procedures.

These procedures have improved how other people respond to me. Every day, strangers and friends tell me they can't believe my age. I enjoy the compliments. In business, doors open that might not have, at least not as easily. The surgeries have also added to the length of my career. When people look tired and aged, it is more difficult to convince others that they are on top of their game. My occupation values vibrancy and health. Cosmetic procedures have prolonged my ability to perform in my chosen field.

I am somewhat open about my surgery. Reactions to discovering my age often require explanation. My facial skin looks younger and less wrinkled than normal for my age. Trying to hide the fact that I have had work done would be like some actresses saying they never had breast implants.

My reluctance to share is that people love to gossip about cosmetic procedures. I had a serious illness and "friends" attributed it to my cosmetic surgery. This hurt because when I needed their support, they implied that vanity caused the illness. There was no connection, but these people were eager to justify their judgment. So I share when I think it is appropriate. If someone is considering a procedure I know about, I am supportive. When people ask me if I have had cosmetic surgery—I always say that I have. If they ask what I've had done, I tell them the things that I choose to. If it is someone I don't want to be specific with, I tell him or her I have had chemical peels or that I have had my eyes done—procedures that are not so controversial. If I feel like being more specific about my surgeries, I am.

Cosmetic surgery is a personal decision and I don't recommend it for everyone. The decision should be based on an honest look at priorities. Personal reflection, motivations, and professional advice should guide the decision. In my reflections, I debated whether I was pursuing the surgery only for vanity. Or whether there was a justification for improving my self -esteem. Attractive people seem to have advantages. I have observed this. Also, Dr. James Dobson says that a child learns as an infant whether he is beautiful or not. For example, people in a grocery store smile at a beautiful child and look away from a child lacking in appearance. He suggests that appearance has an effect on self-esteem, in children and adults. I also know that cosmetic surgery can create a reliance on superficial beauty. While beauty may open some doors, we need to develop our inner selves to be truly successful. Any patient should remember that while beauty has value, it is fleeting no matter what we do. The inner self can be nurtured every day of one's life. I have always looked at it as a bank account. In the beauty bank account, no matter how much I deposit, my account is decreasing annually. In the inner self account, the balance can grow every day.

I also reflected on the opinion of my friends that cosmetic surgery was vain. They took a moral high road saying that they wanted to "age gracefully." They still seemed to pursue improving their appearance and delaying the aging process just as eagerly—only through different means. I can't deny that there is a greater risk in some cosmetic procedures than less invasive ways to improve appearance. But I felt that the risks were low, and the benefits far outweighed the risks.

In assessing motives, the timing of the surgery can be significant. The person may ask, "What event or life circumstance is motivating the procedure at this time?" This answer may reveal how a person expects the outcome to change his or her life. I have known many people with many different reasons for choosing an elective procedure. These run the gamut from seeking improvement with realistic expectations to having delusional beliefs about what a procedure will accomplish.

Motives can also be exposed through the financial commitment. A person's outcome needs to be in balance with the financial sacrifices required. I have seen patients who would sell their souls for one more cosmetic procedure. Surgery addicts are the basis for the criticism that can be directed at healthy patients. Conversely, I have seen patients who had no money and lived with a defect that affected their self-esteem and opportunities every day. (I chose a surgeon who donates his services to these patients on occasion.)

I also strongly considered the motivation of the surgeon. Obviously, a surgeon's income is dependent on surgery. Some doctors perform almost any procedure on a willing, paying customer. It is important to know you're working with a surgeon who is driven by ethics and results more than income. His ethics would prevent him from performing procedures that are not in the best physical or emotional interest of the patient.

Before surgery, I considered the feedback I'd gathered, my motivations and expectations. I meshed those with the professional advice of a trustworthy surgeon. Then I felt prepared to make a qualified decision, a decision I've never regretted.

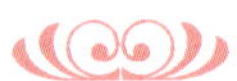

ELIZABETH
The Surgeon's Impressions

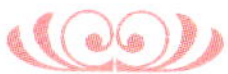

I met Elizabeth and her family approximately twenty years ago when she moved here from the Phoenix area. She is a beautiful woman who worked in the film industry for several years. She came to see me because she had a dorsal kyphosis which is a rather large hump on her nose. That was the one feature that seemed to detract from her appearance. I performed nose enhancement surgery, removing the hump and refining the nasal tip. During the surgery, I also straightened the inside of her nose to improve the airway. Usually after nasal surgery, eighty percent of the swelling is gone in two weeks. Ninety percent of the swelling resolves in two months and an additional one percent of the swelling subsides over a one-year period of time. For patients who have thick skin, it may take up to 18 months for all of the swelling to resolve. In Elizabeth's case, she didn't have thick skin on her nose so her profile was set at about six months.

Nasal procedures are the most difficult surgeries that cosmetic and/or facial plastic surgeons perform. Usually, the first surgery presents the best opportunity for a good result. Revisions (re-operations) are sometimes necessary but I strive to limit them to as few as possible. If you've been in practice as a cosmetic and/or facial plastic surgeon for awhile and you perform nasal surgeries and refinements, you may see patients of other surgeons who need revision. These surgeries can be much more difficult but are just as rewarding as taking a nose that has never been touched either from trauma or surgery and producing the best possible result. My goal is to leave as much of the basic framework of the nose so it is as functional and healthy as possible. I want to make the required modifications necessary to remove a hump on the nose or thin a bulbous tip or reduce wide nostrils, etc. Also, a weak chin can make a person's nose look larger than it actually is: consequently, I like to strengthen the chin with an implant and/or oral surgery. Everything I do is meant to harmoniously balance the profile. But Elizabeth didn't need chin projection, only nasal enhancement.

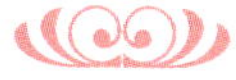

ABIGAIL
Breast Reconstruction

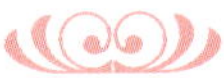

When I was 26 years old, I had to have a mastectomy. Originally, silicone implants were used to reconstruct my breasts, but they certainly did not look normal! I thought I had a good doctor and I'm not saying that I didn't. But with the cosmetic part of the procedure, I'll just say that the doctor didn't care enough. I was very unhappy with the way my breasts looked and I stayed unhappy for years. My breasts never felt like a part of my body and that made me feel inadequate in everything I did, professional or personal. It's strange that a part of my body that no one sees would make me feel so bad. But it did.

Twenty years later, I began to look for a cosmetic surgeon to improve the appearance of my breasts. I had wanted to have something done for at least 10 years but there were two big hurdles. First, I'm very shy about taking my clothes off. Having to show my breasts to another doctor was just devastating. That was so hard for me—just being able to stand in front of someone and say, "Here's what I look like."

Also, the idea of having more surgery troubled me. I wondered if the results would be worth going through another operation. After the mastectomy and reconstruction, I had to have several revision surgeries because of problems with the implants. First, one of the implants ruptured and had to be replaced. Then there was the big scare about silicone implants. So those implants were removed and replaced with saline.

They ruptured too so I had another surgery to replace them with saline implants again. As you can imagine, choosing to have another operation on my breasts was difficult. But I kept thinking that surely enough time had passed that there was a cosmetic surgeon out there who could make me look better.

So I began talking to people who had good cosmetic surgery experiences and one doctor's name kept coming up. I talked to a friend of a surgical nurse about this doctor and she said that all of his patients were treated with complete respect, even when they were asleep. That level of respect was very important to me so I made a consultation appointment.

During my consultation, the doctor told me he could improve the appearance of my breasts but it would take several surgeries. And he recommended silicone implants so they would feel more natural. I was certainly for that! Having had both silicone and saline, I can tell you that there is a huge difference between the two. My first implants were silicone but they didn't feel natural. All of my implants have been placed beneath the muscle because I don't have any breast tissue between my muscle and my skin. But apparently the original implants were positioned in a way that my muscles were strapping them down. My new surgeon had to reposition my chest muscles. I think that contributes to the more natural feel of my breasts now. They not only feel natural but they look natural too.

I've had a total of three revision surgeries with my new surgeon. The first surgery was to maneuver my chest muscles and place silicone implants. But the implants were not large enough. The doctor consulted with the company before my surgery and the surgical rep suggested a certain size. But it was wrong. The only way they could have known the correct size was by seeing inside of me. During the mastectomy, so much tissue was removed that my chest was concave. So the second surgery was to implant a much larger size. In the third surgery, fat was taken from other parts of my body and filled in to give my breasts a better shape. I'm very pleased with the way my breasts look and feel, and I'm through with breast surgery unless an implant ruptures.

My regained confidence affects every part of my life. My career has not only grown but flourished. And I found enough courage to get out of a horrible marriage. The surgeries have changed my entire life by letting me take control.

I would tell those who have a problem with the way they look, "Don't wait as long as I did. Don't let anyone tell you that you're not worth it." But I would advise them to check out their cosmetic surgeon. "Talk to other people, see their results and make sure the surgeon is board certified." In choosing my cosmetic surgeon, I felt good about his credentials and what I'd heard from others, yet when I made my appointment, I was not confident. There's nothing like a personal interview to get a feel for your doctor. When you go for your consultation, you can also check out the atmosphere of the office and the staff. When I walked into the office, I felt the spiritual nature of the people who worked there. My daughter noticed this too when she took me in for surgery. After it was over, I asked her if she was worried. She said, "No, Mom. It didn't even feel like a doctor's office. It was just so calm and peaceful." That's the kind of feeling a patient needs—a sense that the surgeon and staff really care.

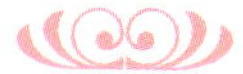

ABIGAIL

The Surgeon's Impressions

This patient had a mastectomy approximately 19 years earlier and was unhappy with the results of several attempts at breast reconstruction. During the mastectomy, tissue was removed very close to the skin so that little tissue between the muscle and the skin remained. Over time, the loss in skin tissue thickness was causing the skin to have an unnatural appearance (dimple) in some areas. Her breasts were asymmetrical—the crease below the left breast was not even with the crease on the right. One breast had more fullness which indicated one of three things: 1) that different size implants were used in the left and right breasts, 2) one implant was slowly leaking, or 3) one breast had less tissue underneath the skin. The latter was the case with Abigail.

One pocket (where the implant was placed) needed to be lowered to increase the symmetry of the breasts. The distance between the bottom of her left breast and the nipple was too long. The lower placement of the implant made the nipple look like a star gazer nipple. (The nipple was positioned above the midline of the breast which made it point up.) There was a concavity of the right breast from the 1 o'clock to the 9 o'clock position. The implants were palpable (could be easily felt) because of the lack of tissue coverage—no breast tissue over her implants. The surgical goal was to improve symmetry and reduce the dimpling. The patient indicated insecurity about how her breasts looked and felt. She was well-proportioned except for her breasts. The challenge was to place the size implant that she needed in order to have breasts that were proportional for her weight and height.

I removed the 350cc saline implants and replaced them with larger silicone implants. She required very large implants (about double what would normally be placed—650 cc.). Before, her breasts looked very small and compressed since she had no significant soft tissue to augment her breast size. The replacement of saline with silicone helped with palpability. I've had to go back and make adjustments because her implants were heavy. The implant stretched her skin because there was no breast tissue integrity. I cut through the capsule that held the implant and folded the tissue on itself so it would be thicker and able to support the implant.

I've filled in areas of her breasts with abdominal fat. Sometimes, putting fat in breasts is considered unacceptable because the fat will calcify and, on mammography, look like little white flecks. These flecks make the radiographer think that cancer may be there when it's not. But since Abigail had the tissue in both of her breasts removed, the use of fat was appropriate. She didn't have much body fat to harvest so I prioritized the areas that received the fat. If she had had more fat, I could have made the breasts look even more natural.

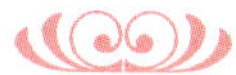

EMILY

Nose Surgery, Eyelid Surgery, Forehead Lift, Fat Transfer and Chemical Peel

I was married for 38 years. To make a long story short, my ex is now married to a 29-years-old. After the divorce, I felt inferior and uncomfortable with myself. Like most women in my situation, I wondered why my husband left. But I also started thinking, "Why not get my nose fixed?" It was something I had always wanted to do. And now, I didn't have anybody to say, "You can't do it." On my dad's side of the family, we have what looks like a ball on the tip of our noses. This is apparent on some people down through the generations. The way mine looked bothered me and I wanted to get it fixed.

So after being divorced for five years, I made appointments with three cosmetic surgeons. After my first consultation, I told my 40-year-old daughter what I was planning. Well, she came unglued! She has been very protective of me since my divorce. She was afraid for my health because I take a blood thinner and would have to get off of the medication before the surgery, then get back on it. I would also have to give myself shots for 10 days before and ten days after the surgery. As a devout Christian, she thought I was being wasteful of my money and vain. But I have lived my whole life for my children and other people. Now I'm 58 years old and at 60, I knew I would look back and wish that I had had my nose fixed.

I finally told her, "I'm not asking you for permission, I am telling you this is what I'm choosing to do. I'm not saying that I'm going to use this doctor or to even pursue this. But it's my decision." I reinforced the fact that I loved her with all of my heart. But this was not about her. My son had a completely different reaction. He said, "Mother, this is your life. Do what you want. Spend your money the way you want to spend it." So having informed both of my children, I was ready for my second appointment.

This appointment was with the doctor who eventually did my surgery. I chose him because he explained every detail—for example, that my skin was thicker than most women's. He also was willing to address my breathing problems. Over the last four years, I had been going to an ear nose and throat specialist because of sinus infections. The specialist had removed some polyps but I still had infections. He told me I needed to do something about them because I couldn't continue the strong antibiotics indefinitely. When I told the cosmetic surgeon about this, he said he didn't know if he could fix these problems but during the surgery, he would see what he could do.

My nose was my priority but I also wanted my eyes done. I've never had a crease in my eyelid: another family trait. At a funeral, I saw a cousin whose eyes are almost closed because of her eyelids. Mine are shaped the same way, so I wondered what my eyes would look like in a few more years. I talked about this issue with the doctor: he agreed that eyelid surgery would be beneficial and recommended a forehead lift as well.

Once I gathered the facts, I made the decision to proceed with the surgery within a couple of months. The cost was a consideration but not a big factor for me. You think you could use the money for other things—like retirement. I always thought this kind of surgery was for people who had lots of money because insurance doesn't cover it. But it's really not that way. I work every day for a living and feel that my surgery was very affordable.

I had two weeks of vacation time coming so scheduling the surgery worked out perfectly for me. I wanted to have my friend come and help me after the surgery and didn't want my daughter to be involved for at least a week. But she said, "Oh no, if you have surgery, I have to be there that day." When she picked me up after surgery, she looked at me and said, "You look like you've been beaten up!" She was not at all prepared for the way I looked. When I got home, I told her to go take care of her children and assured her that everything was fine. Then I called my friend to come over.

After the first 24 hours, my friend went home because I was able to take care of myself. I was surprised that my swelling and bruising were minimal. I am very strong-willed and was determined to follow the post operative instructions exactly as they were written. I think that's why I healed so well. I had a few headaches but they were nothing I couldn't handle. The doctor had said this might happen. The good news is that I haven't even had a sniffle. It's exciting to think about the possibility of having fewer infections as well as a better looking nose.

After two weeks, I went back to work. I told people in my office that I was taking time off to have sinus surgery but didn't tell them about the cosmetic procedures. A few days before returning, I called my office manager and told her what I had done. She said, "You did? I am so interested in this. I would love to have my eyes done." I also called another coworker and said, "I really don't want the whole world to know what I've done but I don't want you to lie about it. Just do what you want with this information." And I just left it like that. When I came back to work, one of my bosses wheeled me around in my chair and said, "Well, let me look." My bosses are psychiatrists. I've worked for them thirteen years. They know about my life and what my marriage was like and have been very supportive.

My family and friends haven't made many comments on my appearance. When my grandchildren saw me they didn't even ask questions. They didn't say that I looked different or ask if I were sick. And you know, children always say whatever they are thinking. I think it's because the way I look now is not a drastic change. I didn't want a drastic change; I just wanted my nose and eyelids to change a little bit and to look a little younger. I see more tightness in my forehead and eyes and my nose is much prettier. Complete healing will take up to a year; swelling goes down very gradually. But I already love the way I feel and look.

I know that my friends like the results too. They are my age and I've gone to church with them through the years. They knew me when I was young and didn't have bags under my eyes. Our children grew up together. They understand and said, "You go first and we'll be right behind you." One friend in particular is very excited about how I healed so quickly and my results. I know that she will be visiting my doctor soon. I will be there to support and take care of her just as she did for me.

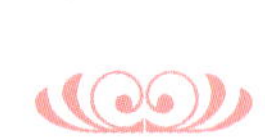

EMILY

The Surgeon's Impressions

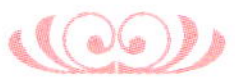

This 58-year-old patient came for a consultation about her eyes and brows. She was also unhappy with her nasal tip. Her eyebrows were attractive and had a nice shape. She plucked them laterally to produce an arch at a perpendicular angle from the lateral limbus (side of the pupil) straight up. This arch creates a very pretty eyebrow for women. However, her eyes appeared sad even though she had a lovely demeanor and personal charm. The significant amount of extra skin on her upper eyelids, sagging skin in her mid-brow area and lateral hooding (covering of skin on the side of the eyes) all contributed to the extra skin over her upper eyelashes. She needed to have a brow lift as well as an upper blepharoplasty (eyelid surgery) in order to give her eyes a more youthful, open look. One other feature of importance was that she had a high forehead. So I couldn't afford to raise it any higher. That meant that the brow lift needed to be performed through an incision at the hairline. This approach doesn't raise the hairline and possibly lowers it a few millimeters.

Emily also had some pseudoherniated fat in her lower eyelid compartments (bags and puffiness below the eyes). This fat created bulges or bags below her eyes. The fat below the eye is made up of small lobules and needs to be removed. The incisions are made on the inside of the cul-de-sac of the conjunctiva (the inside of the lower eyelids). Once that fat is removed, fat is taken from the abdomen and centrifuged (spun) to produce a slurry (a watery substance with suspended fat particles). I smooth the area beneath the eyes by injecting the slurry into it. Some doctors don't advocate the removal of the existing fat below the eyes. They just inject the slurry in and around it. My concern is that if the slurry is absorbed by the body, the patient reappears with the bags and says, "Doctor, I paid you to take these bags out and now they're back." If the fat is absorbed, a little more fat is added to take care of the situation.

The descent of the fat in Emily's mid-face created indentions along her orbital rims (the bones around the outer edge of her eyes). Some of the fat that was taken from the abdomen was injected into this area as well as the upper cheeks to fill them out. I followed the injection of fat with a chemical peel on the skin around the eyes. The peel tightened the tissue and contributed to a more youthful look. These procedures avoid lid retraction which is the pulled down or stark, staring eye look. Lower eyelid retraction often results from the traditional lower eyelid blepharoplasty (eyelid surgery) when an incision is made just underneath the lower lash line.

Emily's bulbous nose tip was corrected with a tip-plasty (reshaping the end of the nose). The tip was not anything of great magnitude but she felt it made her look more masculine.

All of these procedures – the eyelid rejuvenation, brow lift, fat transfer, chemical peel and nasal tip plasty were performed at the same time. Emily's healing process was uneventful and each time she returned for follow up she was happier than the time before. It's important for patients to understand that the healing process takes place gradually over a period of weeks and months. The final results may not be apparent for up to six months.

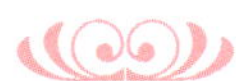

KATHERINE
Body Lift

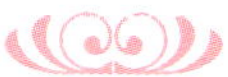

I was getting older and had saggy skin around my thighs and buttocks. I didn't want to look old; I was just not ready for that yet! I had been thinking about doing something about this part of my body for a couple of years. I just didn't know when it would happen. Then, the man I loved was killed. I had a really tough time for a year before I finally went into therapy. I was having physical symptoms (digestive problems) as a result of my grief so my doctor recommended a therapist. The therapist told me I needed to do something for myself. And that was all I needed. I knew it was time to call my cosmetic surgeon.

In the late 80s or early 90s, my sister had used a surgeon to repair her nose. She learned about him through someone who had been his patient. Since that time other members of my family, some of my friends and my clients have used him for various procedures. My mother just had a facelift. She's 68 years old and now looks like my sister. Several years ago, he had performed an upper and lower eyelid surgery for me. I was very pleased with the difference it made. There are many cosmetic surgeons in my area of the state, but my positive experiences keep me coming back to this one.

I had not lost much weight. I've always been thin but I didn't look good in a bathing suit and I wanted to. This surgery was the way to reach that goal. I was not anxious. It was really a simple procedure for me. I didn't realize until later that it was major surgery because I was never in any pain. When I woke up my mother said, "Why didn't you tell me this was major surgery? I can't believe you did this!" I was uncomfortable from time to time, especially during the first 72 hours. But the doctor and nurses made sure that I had no pain. The surgery was done at a hospital and I stayed one night, then released to go home which is three hours away. My mom stayed with me a couple of days until I could take care of myself. I borrowed my grandmother's "grabber" to reach things because I couldn't bend over for a while after the surgery. My mother brought me back for the first couple of follow up visits because I couldn't drive. But after that, I drove myself.

This surgery has improved my self-esteem. It helped me recover from the grief. I just have a better feeling about myself and I project that to everyone around me. I know surgery can't stop the aging process but it definitely can set it back a few years. I would have a body lift again in a minute. I didn't need to lose weight but I had cellulite in my rear and it looked like hail damage. I'm not heavy but that was just the type of skin I had. When I explain my surgery, people look at me like I'm crazy. They think it really hurt. But it didn't. I can't think of any negative aspects to my experience. I highly recommend this surgery for anyone who's lost a lot of weight or someone like me who just has baggy, saggy issues. I think this is the surgery of the future because more people are finding out about it. All of my clients who know I've had a body lift say, "I did not know that could be done." One client who had bariatric surgery and lost about a hundred pounds in a year says she definitely wants to have the surgery because of the extra skin.

I'm very open with others about my surgery because many people don't know this type of procedure is available. But I'm very clear that they must find the right surgeon. Many people who are not board certified perform cosmetic surgery. It's very important to do your research. If you are considering a particular surgeon, talk to someone who has used them for that specific surgery. It always helps to talk to someone who has been through it.

Most of my clients know about my surgery because I went back to work after ten days. I had ordered some yoga pants that I wore with a long tunic because I had to wear a compression garment for six weeks. It's best to have the surgery in the winter or early spring so healing occurs before it gets hot. My surgery was scheduled for March 8th and I had a wedding to attend on the 17th. I was leaving for the beach on May 19th. So I wanted to heal quickly.

My best advice about recovery is to follow all of the surgeon's instructions. Don't do the things the surgeon tells you not to do. That is so very important. When he tells you, "I want you to do this or I don't want you to do that," there is a reason for it. Here are some other tips for people who have a body lift. Be sure to wear the ointment and the tape. Use baby wipes (or something similar) because they are soothing. Be good to yourself during the healing process. And one last thing, I asked the surgeon to make the incision underneath my thong underwear so it would hide the scars and it does! I'm very pleased with the limited amount of scaring that I have.

I still want to have liposuction on some of the fat around my thighs but the surgeon said I need to wait a year for my body to heal. I really respect that because if you remove too much fat, it's really hard to replace it. I would love for him to do my nose. I see myself as a work in progress. I am definitely a repeat offender.

KATHERINE

The Surgeon's Impressions

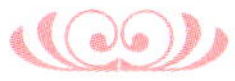

This 48-year-old client came to see me about two years after experiencing a tragic loss. Katherine is a thin woman, but was unhappy with the dimpled appearance of her thighs as well as her buttocks. She had little or no fat to be removed. Her biggest issue was the loss of skin elasticity. I felt that the best option for Katherine was a body lift. This lift would entail not only lifting the buttocks and the side and front of each thigh, but the middle portion of the upper leg as well. Body lift is performed under general anesthesia with as little as one or two days of hospital stay. The thigh as well as the buttock area is improved by removing skin above those areas as well as the skin in the flank and lower abdomen.

Katherine tolerated this procedure quite nicely and healed well. Her best improvement is in her buttock region, where she has a nice lift with good posterior projection. She also has a good result in the medial (middle) thigh area where I removed two to three inches of skin in the crease above the groin. The removal of this skin improves the upper one-third of the medial (middle) thigh. I removed 4½ to 5 inches of skin from the lateral (outside) thigh which tightens the upper one half of this area of the leg. In doing these procedures, you cannot put tension on the skin during the repair so that is why it's called a high tension lateral thigh lift. You are actually suturing the soft tissue of the lower leg at a higher level to the fascial layers (inside tissue) of the upper trunk. This type of suturing prevents little or no stretch back so you don't lose the improvement you gain during the surgical procedure. Body lift is a relatively simple (but lengthy) procedure, especially if the patient has no chronic disease issues. However, the surgery does leave incisional body scars. They fade over time (6-24 months). Sometimes it is necessary to perform minor revision procedures if the patient has problems associated with healing. Katherine requested that I place the incisions so that the scars would be covered by thong underwear. She seems very pleased with the location of her scars as well as the results of her surgery.

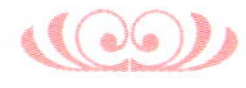

MARY

Breast Surgery (Lift and Augmentation)

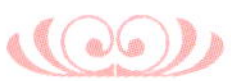

Before my surgery, I didn't want to take off my shirt in front of my husband. I wanted to be intimate with him only in the dark. I trust my husband totally and am blessed with a wonderful marriage. But this wasn't about our relationship. It was about me and what I saw through his eyes when we were together. My feelings started to be a burden and led to my decision to have breast enhancement surgery.

But I must think about the breast enhancement in connection with my gastric bypass. Bypass surgery helped me lose almost a hundred pounds in about a year. I wasn't a fat kid. I became very hungry after I married. I ate nutritious food—but a lot of it. For years, I tried to lose weight on my own and just couldn't do it. This was defeating, depressing and upsetting. After I lost the weight, my stomach looked okay and the rest of my body looked okay too. I looked like I was 40 years old, which I am. I'm okay with looking my age but I felt like my breasts looked 80 years old. I was not okay with that. The rest of my body looked healthy and strong but that one part of me didn't. Regardless of the exercises I tried, that part of my body did not respond.

The decision to have the bypass was huge. Compared to that decision, breast surgery was a little one. I visited one other cosmetic surgeon before my consultation with this doctor. Then I visited another one after. The first doctor said I needed a breast lift and he didn't do them, only implants. A friend who had implants to correct a severe asymmetry in her breasts recommended another surgeon. This surgeon had done reconstructive breast surgery and said, "Oh, I think we can do the lift and the implants at the same time. You're borderline but I think we can do it all at once." Financially, that was a benefit – only one surgery instead of two. But the doctor I chose said, "I don't think you'll be happy if we do it as one surgery." The more I thought about it, the more I wanted to go with his more conservative approach.

I got serious about breast surgery about a year before having it done. The delay wasn't because I was uncomfortable with the idea; it was because some big life events came up. Surgery had to go on the back burner for a while. There was a bit of a financial hurdle too. Also, I had to work out some concerns; how to care for my two and a half year-old son and how my family would react.

I felt pretty badly about using so much of our financial resources for what seemed to boil down to my vanity. They're just breasts. Why are they so important to me? On the other hand, we had the money and our bills were getting paid. Overall, my husband and I are both happy about how the money was spent. I didn't have anyone to help with child care after the surgery, and when my son wanted his Mama, I needed to be there for him. So we worked out a way for my little guy to climb in and out of the tub and he could climb into his car seat by himself. I would get down in the floor and he could climb into my lap. We're still using many of these adaptations because they let him be more independent. My family was supportive of my breast lift but without exception said, "Well, just so long as you're not getting implants!" So when it came time to get implants, I decided not to tell them.

My breast surgery was done in two stages. I had the lift first so the scars from the surgery would have a chance to heal. Immediately after the lift, I had some swelling and thought my breasts were perfect. I didn't need implants. But the swelling lasted only a few weeks. Still, my breasts were in a position they had never been before. I really liked that when I leaned over they didn't just hang down any more. Once, before my surgery, I was washing my face without a bra and my husband came into the bathroom. I quickly covered myself up. I just felt like my breasts were hanging there like udders!

Five months after the breast lift, I had the implants. Originally, the doctor suggested waiting six months to a year between the breast surgeries. But I healed so well he said we could go ahead. When I chose the volume of the implants, it was hard to get comfortable with the size. It was a tough decision because everything looked too big. I thought everybody would be staring at me and I don't like that kind of attention. But the nurse was very patient with me. We started trying out small ones and then worked up to larger sizes. She kept saying, "I think you'll wish you had gone larger." It's hard to imagine what the implants will look like once they're under your muscle. Before my breast surgery, I felt like a walking set of hips and a rib cage—very out of balance. So when I tried on the implants I thought I looked like a walking set of breasts. First I tried on the 300 cc and said, "Oh, no." Then I tried the 325 cc and said, "No way!" At 350 cc I thought, "This is as much as I can tolerate." I asked the nurse what size the doctor recommended after he measured me. She said, "375 cc." I remembered when he measured me, he kept saying, "You've got to balance out your hips." So I tried on the 375 cc and my husband said, "Oh Mary, that's it!" The nurse said that when the implants were inside my body they would look more like the 350s looked when I tried them on. So then my husband said, "Try the 400s!"

But I made the decision to go with the 375 cc implants. My thinking was that this doctor had done many of these surgeries and knew what he was talking about. The nurse assured me that he would discourage getting implants that were too large for my body structure. And the doctor was right. If I had gone smaller I wouldn't be as happy as I am now. If my breasts were any larger, I would be in a D cup and I don't want that. I'm a medium size girl and want a medium size cup. I understand that many women wish they had chosen a larger size but I'm very satisfied. I never look down and think I wish I'd gone bigger. I did look at a picture of myself with clothes on before the breast surgery. I don't look any different now because, at that time, I just had extra skin and I wore a bra on top of it. My breasts just hung around in the bottom of the bra. Of course the cups were really stiff so it worked.

I thought my family wouldn't notice the implants, but they did. I was anxious about telling them but in the long run, I think I did it the best way. I had the implants in early May and had my whole family visit Memorial Day weekend. I was nervous about what they would think. I had long hair before the surgery and had it cut much shorter before they came. I hoped they would focus on my hair instead of my breasts. But they noticed both!

I am not completely open about my surgery. I can't stand the idea that someone might think of it in a negative way. For example, I don't want people at work to gossip about me. On the other hand, I don't mind telling the people who are my friends, who wouldn't be gossiping. I told a group of friends about my breast lift but when I decided to have implants, I didn't say anything. I thought they might think I was some sort of surgery addict. I'm not ashamed of my decision. I just don't want people to talk about it. I don't want to be the woman who got breast implants. I don't want to be defined by my surgery. I want to be defined by my good or bad characteristics, like my sense of humor.

I wouldn't recommend cosmetic surgery to anyone who thought it would change her life from bad to good. I'm really glad I had my surgery but I still have the same life. I didn't want to change that. The surgery just helped me feel more positive about myself. I like what I see in the mirror. When I lost the weight, I looked better and was healthier. But the best part was that I didn't think about my weight any more. When you're overweight, you spend all of your energy thinking about it. Maybe everybody doesn't, but I did. I thought that being heavy was all people saw and all they would remember about me. Then, after my weight loss, I was free from all of that. Likewise, when I enhanced my breasts, I stopped thinking about them. When I get dressed, I make sure I look okay but I don't think about it the rest of the day.

I also have more confidence in the intimate part of my marriage. Because I'm more comfortable and confident, I'm more interested in our sex life. That's been a positive development for my husband too. I read that most women report an increased sex drive after having implants and thought that was silly. But sex is more interesting when you're not worried about what he sees. I knew that what he was seeing was just me and that he thought I was beautiful. He told me that all of the time. But I wanted to feel as beautiful as he thought I was.

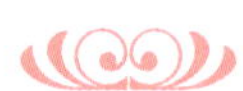

MARY

The Surgeon's Impressions

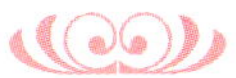

Mary lost a large amount of total body weight as a result of gastric bypass surgery. Many women who lose significant body mass tend to lose volume in their breasts. When some patients—particularly young ones—lose volume, their skin contracts. But in Mary's situation, her tissue had lost its elastic properties, leaving an empty skin envelope that needed to be filled and also lifted. She had loose skin that needed to be removed. Also, breast tissue that had fallen onto her upper abdomen needed to be repositioned and contoured in a more desirable shape. Mary and I discussed a two-pronged surgical approach in order to minimize the scarring of her breasts. The first surgery would remove the loose skin, re-contour the breast into a more conical form and reposition it higher on the chest wall. The second surgery, approximately six months later and after the initial scars were healed, would be to insert breast implants to create a bust line that was proportional to the rest of Mary's body.

The first surgery that I performed on Mary was a vertical mammoplasty utilizing a "lollipop incision." It is performed in order to lift breasts, to shape breasts and/or to reduce breast size. In Mary's situation, I needed to position the nipple-areolar complex (the nipple and surrounding areola) higher on the chest wall at approximately 20 centimeters from the base of the neck. This placement is crucial for a good result because the implants are positioned dead center behind the nipple. If you don't raise the nipple up on the chest wall, then you have a breast that's much too low and doesn't look right. I did not remove any breast tissue but re-contoured the existing tissue into a more appropriate shape. As a result, Mary's breasts were basically the same size but at a higher level on her chest wall. After five months, I performed the second surgery to place 375 cc silicone implants under her chest wall muscle. This sub muscular placement was ideal for Mary because she had very little breast tissue to cover the implants.

I help patients determine the size of their implants based on age, body morphology (shape), height, width of the chest, size of the hips, size of the abdomen, and sometimes, lifestyle. I try to individualize the breast shape with all those parameters and more taken into account. In Mary's case she had lost a large amount of weight, but was still a moderate framed woman in her early forties. I wanted to give her a nice, robust size but not overload her. Large implants can make a short person look dowdy or matronly. Tall, thin women can usually handle bigger breast implants. Also, the morphology or shape of the implants has a lot to do with the result so I discuss these issues with patients.

Before the surgeries, Mary was a deflated "A" cup. Now she is a full, perky "C" cup. The last time Mary was in the office, she was thrilled with her results. Her incisional scars are healing very well. She said she was glad she did the two-pronged approach because, in the end, the scars are less noticeable. All in all, Mary is happy with her breasts size, position and their shape. It has made her much more self-confident both at home and with the public.

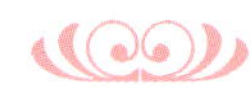

NATALIE

*Liposuction, Eyelid Surgery, Forehead Lift, Facelift, Chin Implant, Nose Surgery,
Earlobe Reduction, Fat Transfer, Dermabrasion and Chemical Peel*

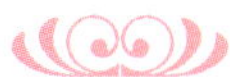

I already had a terrific life—a wonderful husband, family, friends and career. So I would never say that cosmetic surgery made me happy. I would say that it was the icing on the cake. Before my surgery, I would look in the mirror each morning and think: "Did I get any rest at all?" I looked just like I did when I went to bed the night before—exhausted. I felt exhausted too. I love my career but it's very stressful. As an interior designer, I spend a great deal of energy on my clients. I look for the threads in their lives and pull them together to create a unique space. Sometimes it feels like my clients own me. I work weekends as well as weekdays.

I always thought that I would like to have cosmetic surgery, so when I had the opportunity to have a makeover, I jumped at the chance. The patient liaison in a cosmetic surgeon's office knew the doctor was looking for a makeover patient. He wanted someone who had some name recognition and would be easy to talk to; someone who would answer questions from the public without hesitation. The liaison suggested that the doctor and I meet. The next thing I knew, I was in this whirlwind of activity; meeting doctors and arranging schedules. Everything was filmed for TV so my experience was never private.

My makeover was more a process than a single event. First I went on a diet and began exercising. I had to lose weight because the initial procedure was liposuction on my midsection. I made the lifestyle changes, dieting and exercising, to be healthier so my recovery would be easier. Also, the lifestyle changes helped me feel better about myself and relieved some stress.

Right after the liposuction, I had a dental makeover. Then seven months after the liposuction, I had cosmetic surgery on my face. This surgery included a full facelift, a chin implant, earlobe reduction, nasal refinement and eyelid and skin rejuvenation. Before the surgery, I asked the doctor if he wanted me to bring some old photographs of myself. He said he didn't need them. He is very talented. It's like he looks inside you and sees your beauty. He doesn't try to make you look like somebody else—just restore your youthfulness. I trusted the doctor completely and my husband was so well informed that I was never worried. I just showed up and enjoyed the whole process. The doctor's office arranged for a trainer, a hair colorist, and someone to help me with makeup. It was just an extraordinary Cinderella kind of experience.

I've truly enjoyed sharing my makeover. Video of my surgery was aired to the public and my experience appeared in many magazines. Because of this, people felt free to come up and ask questions. I was at a furniture market in Dallas and a woman came up to me and said, "I know who you are!" It's been fun and rewarding to give confidence to other women who want to have something done. I tell these women that if it's something you want and you have someone to take care of you, go ahead. I always recommend that they make sure they're in the right doctor's hands. The ultimate decision is who's going to do the surgery. You've got to have someone with expertise and someone in whom you have a high level of trust. It's also important to get a doctor who'll be available to you after you go home.

I can get very emotional about my surgery and the doctor. I learned so much about gifts and talents. This doctor was given a talent and chooses to bless others with it. I won't say that the surgery changed my life because I don't want anyone to think that cosmetic surgery will assure happiness. But what the doctor does is life-giving because it enhanced my life in many ways. Every person in his office cares. Their interest in my well-being was one of the most loving experiences I have had. There was pain in the makeover process but there was more love than anything else.

Through this process, I also learned about my husband's love for me. I knew Michael loved me, but I had no idea about the depth of his love. I will never forget it. We spent the first night in a hotel because we live out of town. When the doctor came to check on me that night he said, "Natalie, we've never had a husband who is as efficient and loving as yours." Michael had a table set up with the medicines and a piece of paper under each one that listed the times to take it. He was on top of everything so I was confident I would be okay.

Michael wouldn't let me look at myself for the first few days, so I knew I had to look scary. I was taking showers several times a day and he would guide me into the shower past the mirror so I couldn't see. When I saw myself for the first time, I couldn't believe it. I thought I looked like I had been in a car wreck. Michael said, "You look great. You have no idea how you looked before!"

We slept in two recliners for at least two weeks. Michael never got up to go to bed. I'd wake up sometimes and not be aware that I was making noises. There he would be, on one knee, rubbing my hand, saying, "It's okay, go back to sleep." Or I'd wake up and look over at him sleeping. He was there all of the time. I didn't think our relationship could get stronger, but it did.

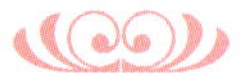

MICHAEL

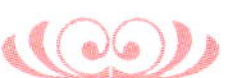

Natalie and I have always been close. We love being able to share experiences; cosmetic surgery was one of those. I was hesitant when we first started considering the makeover, especially when I started watching facelifts on the medical channel. I would watch for just a few minutes and turn it off. I just couldn't take it. But I kept going back and watching the show until I understood the surgery from the beginning to the end. When we finally made the decision to have the makeover, I knew what to expect. But seeing surgery on TV and having your wife go through it is very different. When you're watching TV, you're seeing someone you don't know. All of that changes when it happens to the woman you adore. You know it's going to be painful.

I'll never forget when they brought Natalie out after surgery. She was in a wheelchair. Her head was all bandaged up so she really couldn't see me. But I knew she was concerned about how I felt because she was waving her hand saying, "I'm okay, I'm okay."

After the surgery, I made sure Natalie took her medicines and showers on time. I treated her stitches. Having me there made it easier on her. I was lucky to be able to have the time to care for her and would recommend that patients have someone there for up to two weeks if necessary. I knew that everything was going to be okay because I trusted the doctor and knew what to expect. Also, the doctor's office was in touch with me every day. The nurses called and the doctor called. If I became concerned, they were there to answer my questions. It has all been worth it to see Natalie so happy. She meets the public every day so it's important for her to feel good about herself.

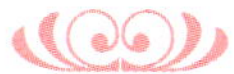

NATALIE

The Surgeon's Impressions

When the makeover shows were popular, I was asked to perform a facial rejuvenation for a national audience. The host of the show worked with my office, agreeing to videotape Natalie before, during and after her surgery. Natalie was selected because she is a well-known interior designer having worked in homes all over the country. I wanted her personality to be reflected in her appearance because she's such a young-hearted, vivacious person.

Because she has a round face, Natalie needed to lose weight in order to maximize the change in her before and after pictures. A round face usually doesn't show as much improvement from facial rejuvenation as a more angular face. Losing weight helps to reduce facial fullness, creating a more angular appearance. To jumpstart the weight loss, I agreed to do liposuction on her abdomen and, in February, I extracted almost five liters of fat tissue. She continued her weight reduction program and lost over 30 pounds by the time she had facial surgery in September.

Natalie received a complete facial rejuvenation. I placed a chin implant in conjunction with a lower facelift, liposuction around the jaw line, dermabrasion to help improve the lines around her mouth and a brow lift. She has a high forehead so I placed the incision for the lift at the hairline so as not to raise it. Natalie has beautiful blue eyes that seem to show her soul so I wanted to highlight this feature. I performed upper and lower eyelid surgery, removed the fat from under her lower lids and chemically peeled the skin to tighten it. I placed some fat along her upper cheek area and her lips to enhance their fullness.

In addition, Natalie's earlobes were reduced. One of the problems of aging is long, torn or creased earlobes. Earlobes that are too fleshy, long or low just don't go with a face that's been rejuvenated. So I implore many of my patients who have this condition and are getting a facelift to allow me to reduce their earlobes. Sometimes, I remove 50-80% because the lobe is stretched so far. I detach the earlobe from the side of the face when I'm beginning the facelift. Then I cut the fleshy part of the earlobe from back to front and remove a wedge. I recreate the curve in the bottom of the earlobe and bunch the earlobe up on the side of the face to reattach it. When the face heals after facelift surgery and the skin begins to relax, the skin tends to drag the earlobe down and can create a "pixie" ear. To avoid that, I bunch the earlobe up, taking future skin relaxation into account. Sometimes, I have to cut out the pierced earring holes that exist and re-pierce them after they've healed in six weeks to three months.

Conservatively, Natalie looks 10 to 12 years younger as a result of these cosmetic procedures. Her after pictures don't reflect the 30-pound weight loss since I moved the tissue in her face back to a more youthful position and filled in the areas that were sunken. That's why she has the facial fullness in the after picture. After she lost weight in her face, she had more facial sag. But she still had enough volume that once I got the fat deposits back into position and added a little more fat, her face looked less gaunt and much more lifted and rested.

The whole experience with Natalie and Michael was fun. They were troopers throughout the whole process. Natalie recovered from the surgery very well and looks great. A lot of that was her doing. She lost the weight and had the unwavering support of her husband. These factors contributed to her ultimate outcome.

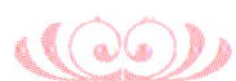

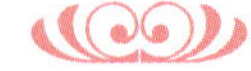

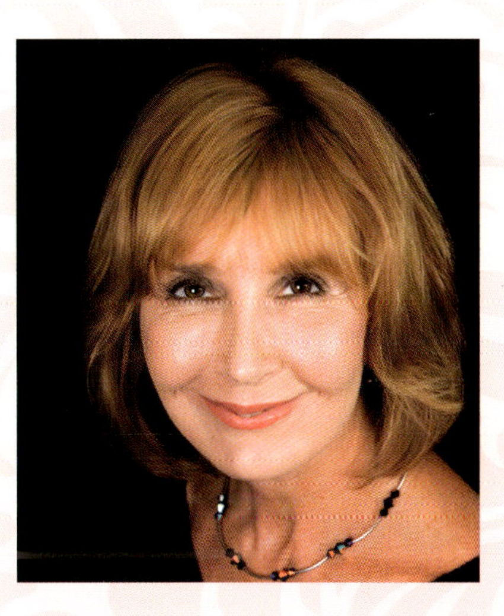

AMAZING TRANSFORMATIONS

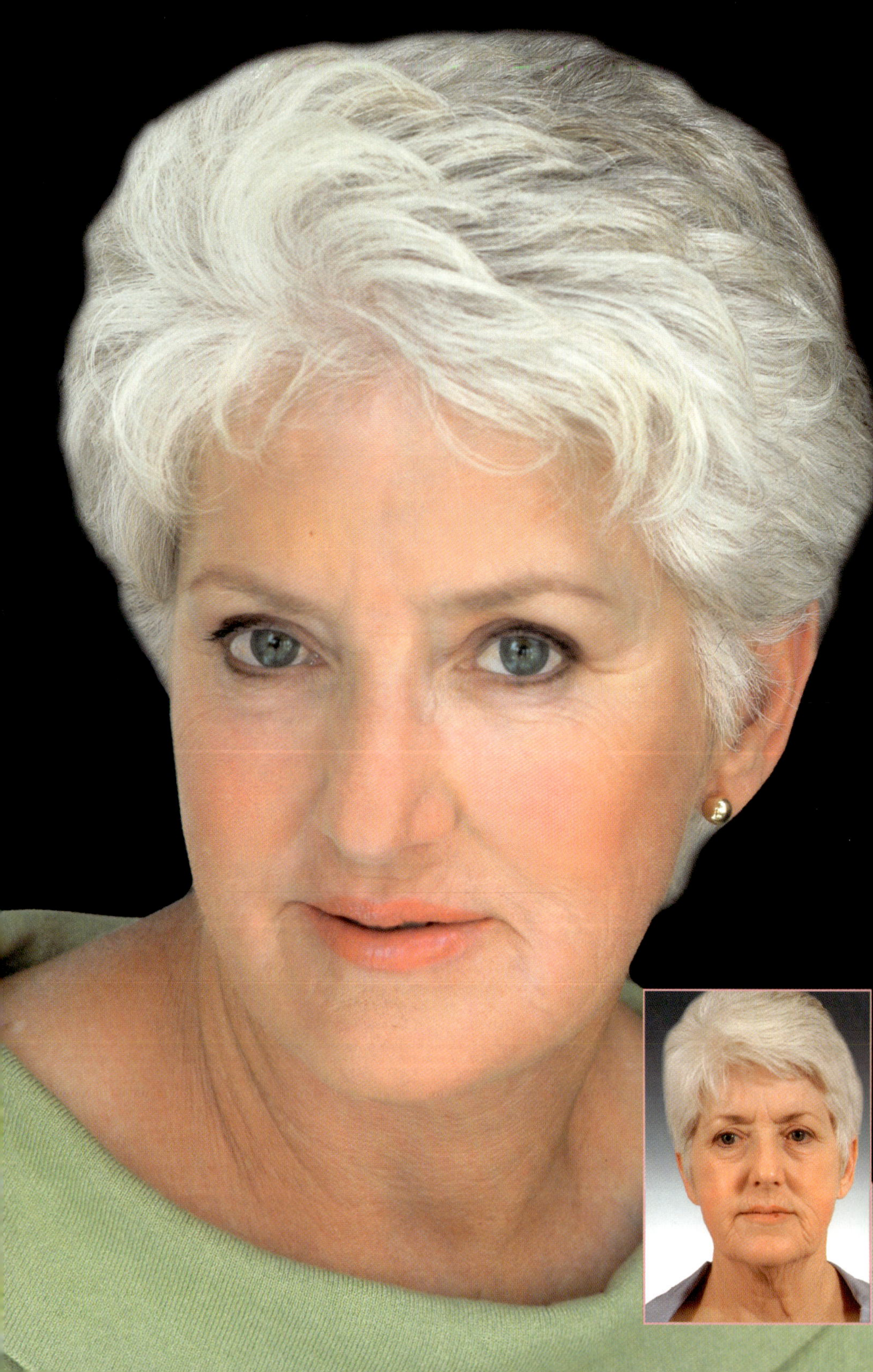

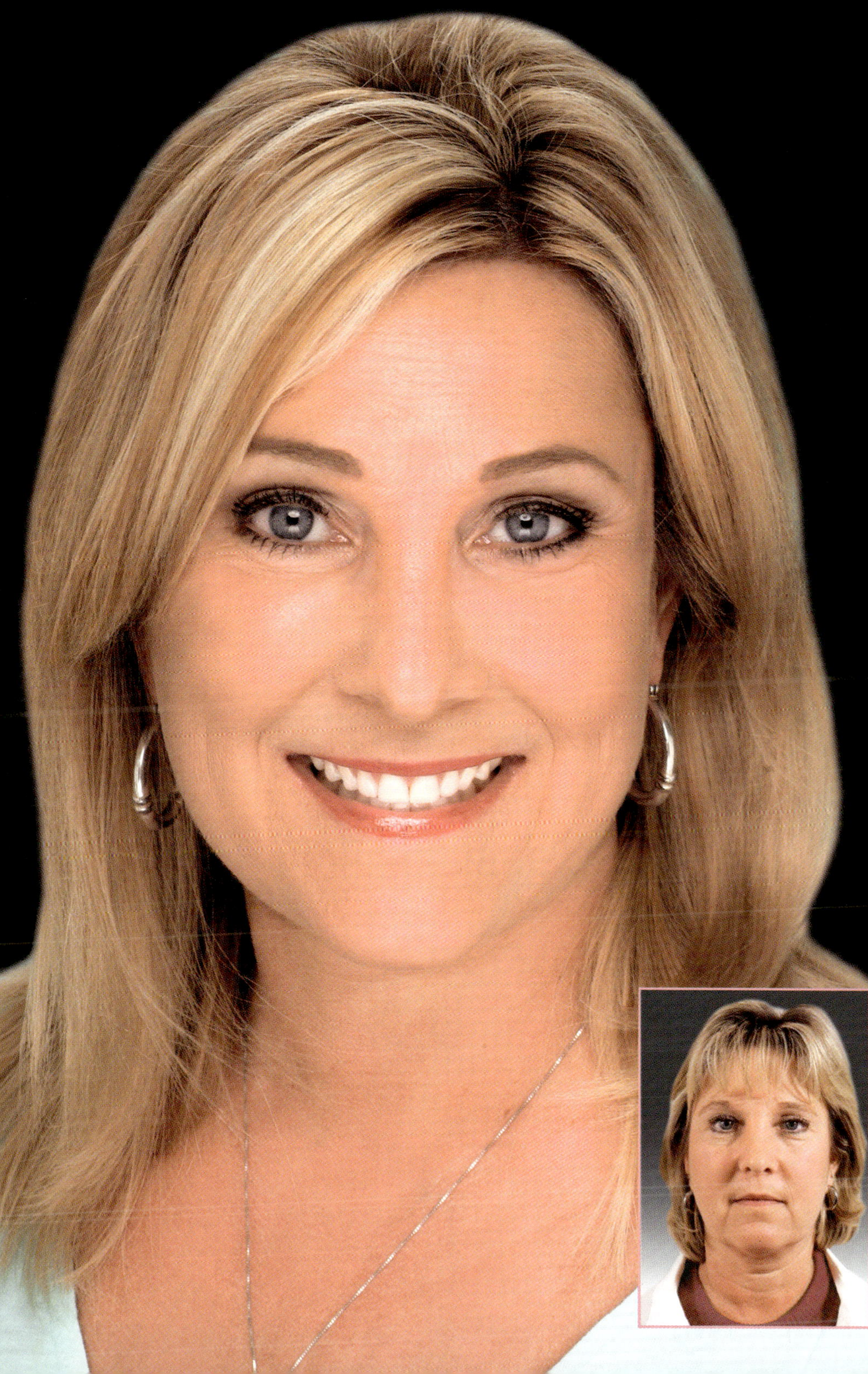

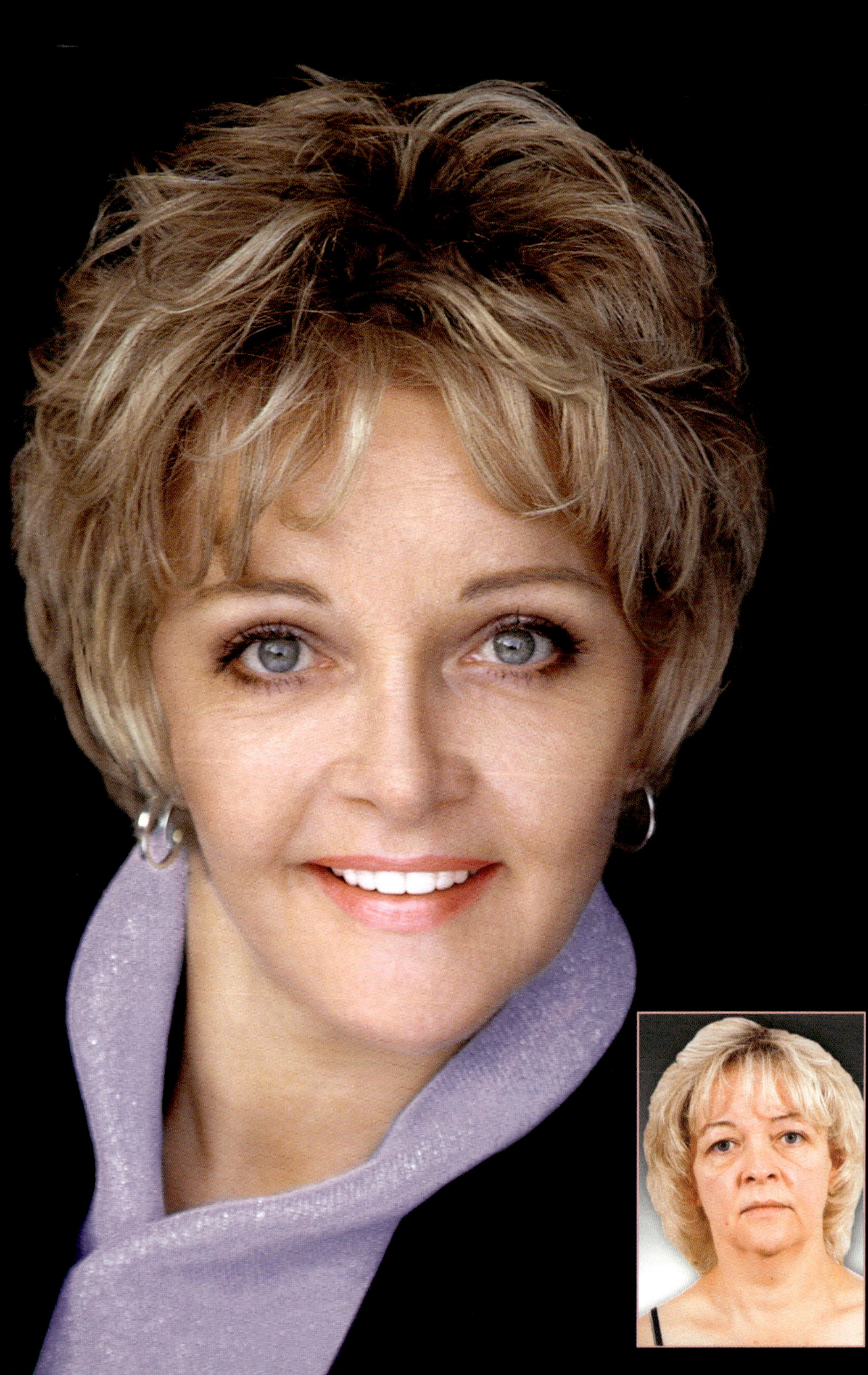

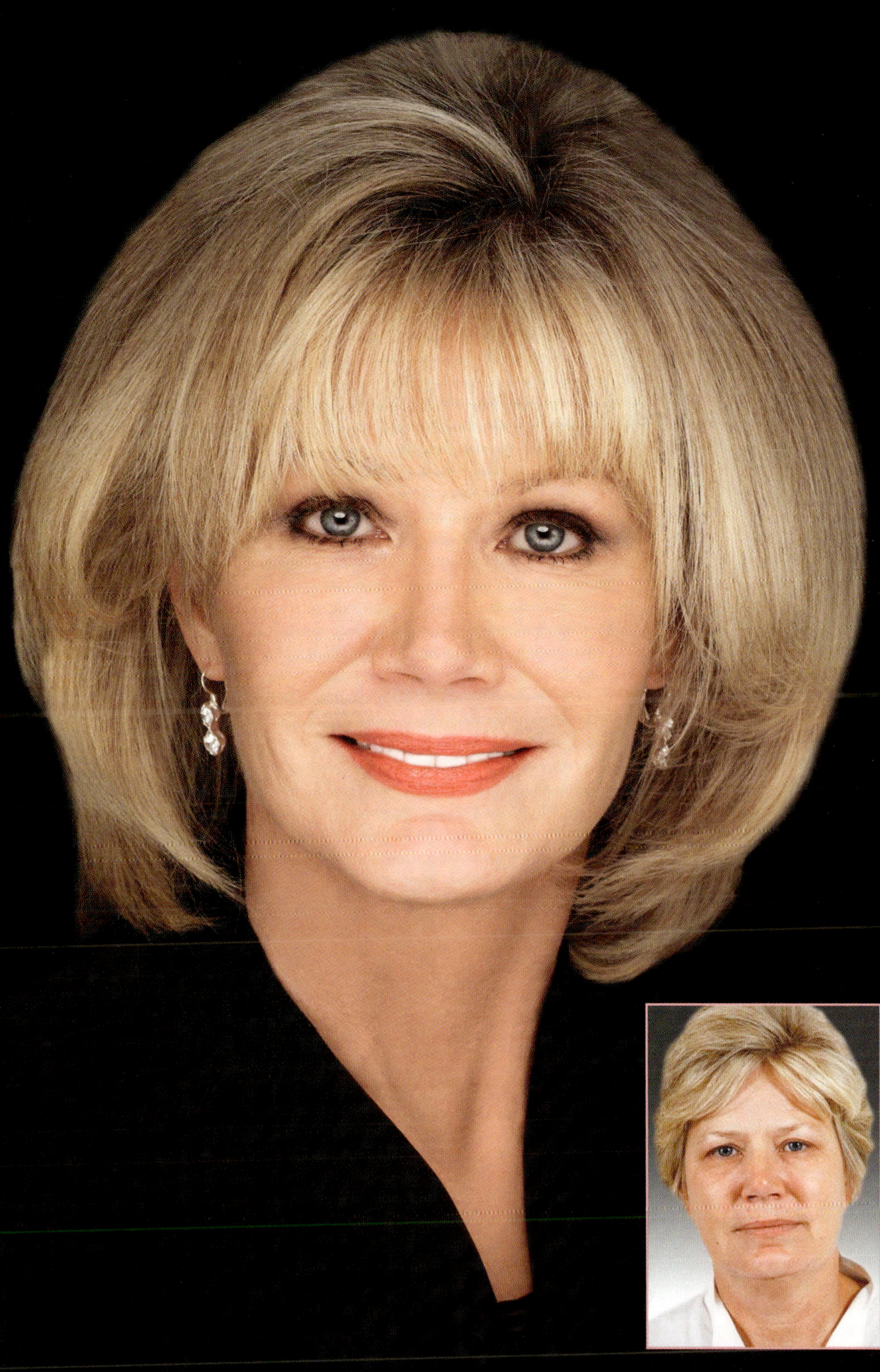

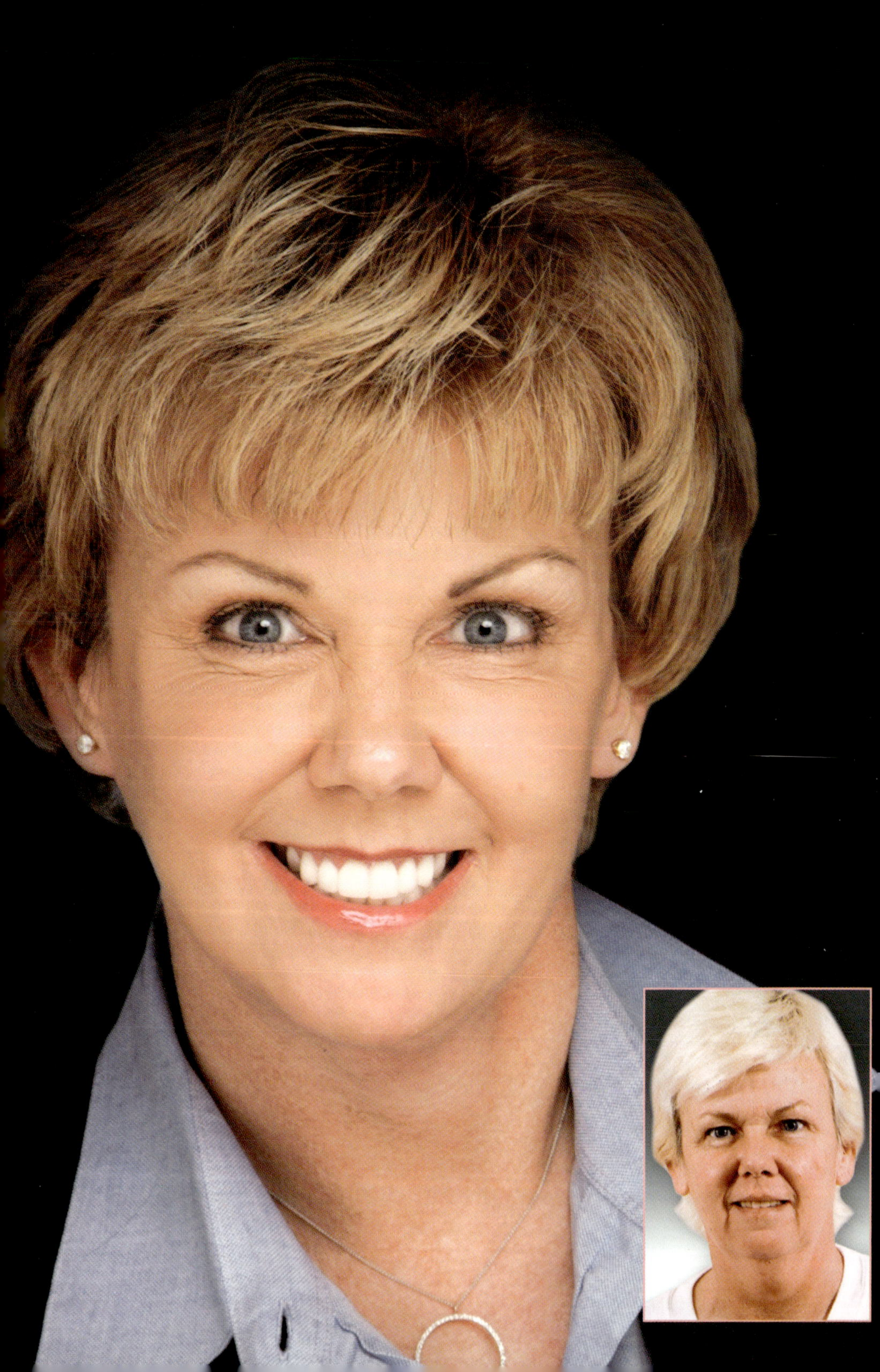

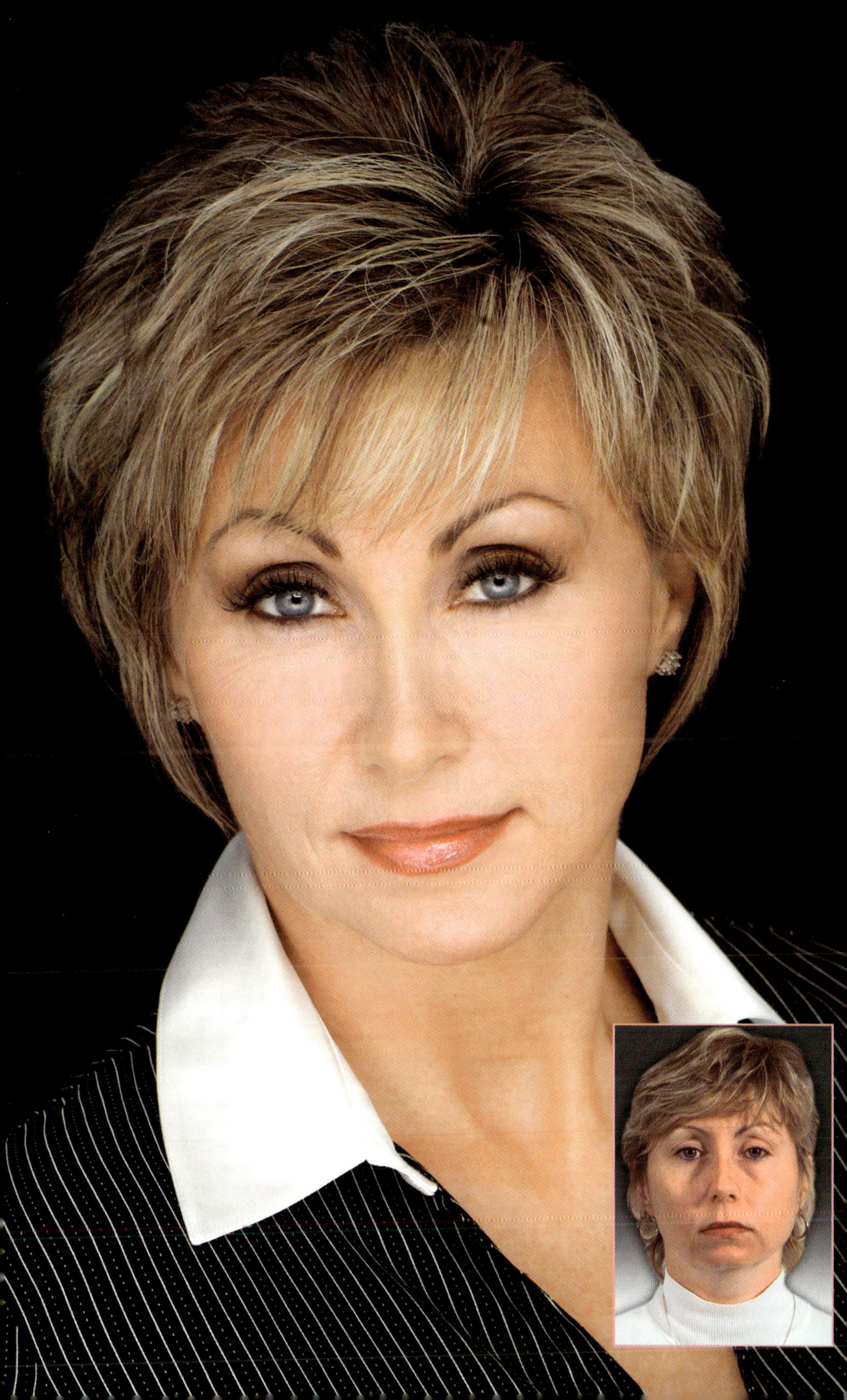

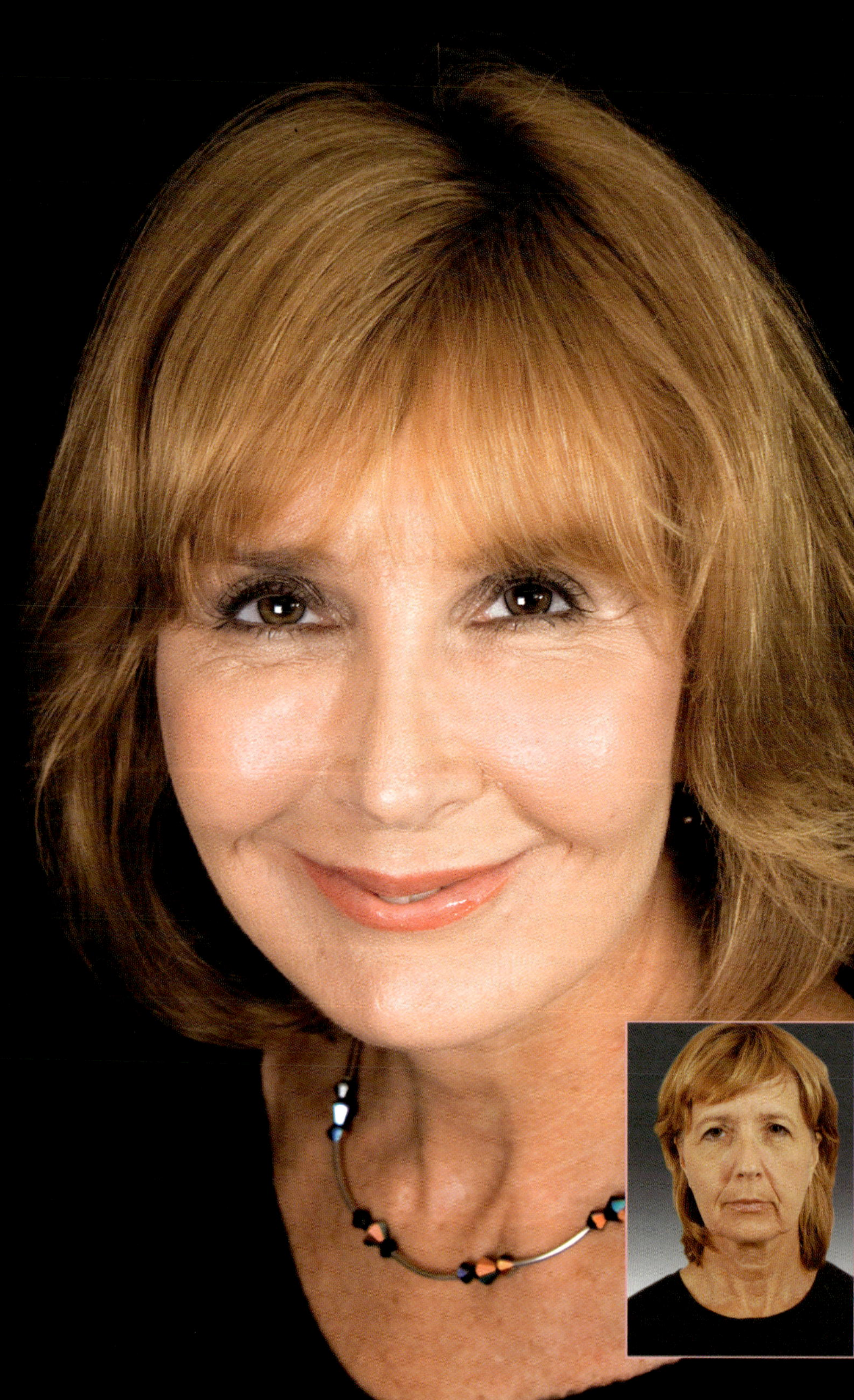

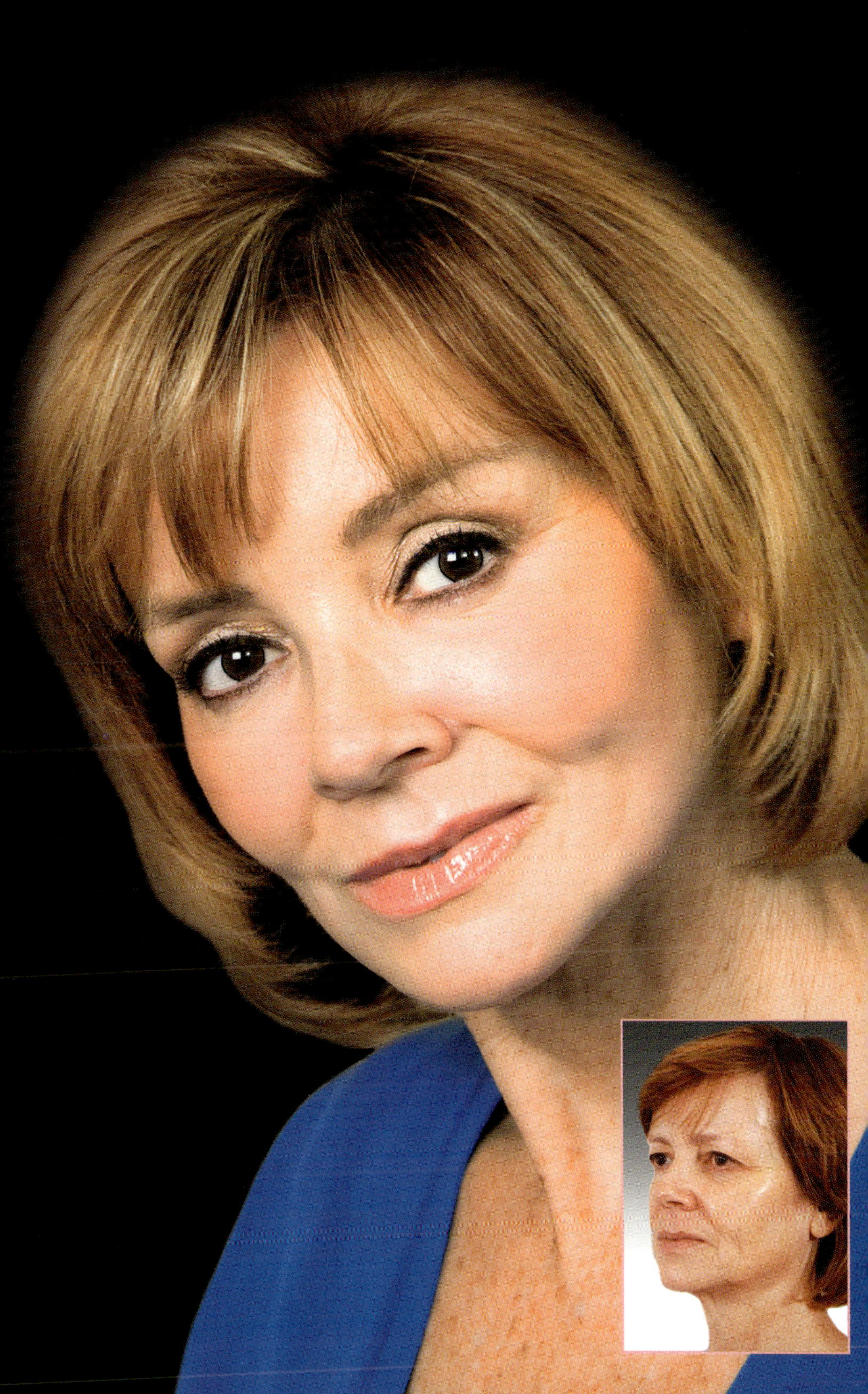

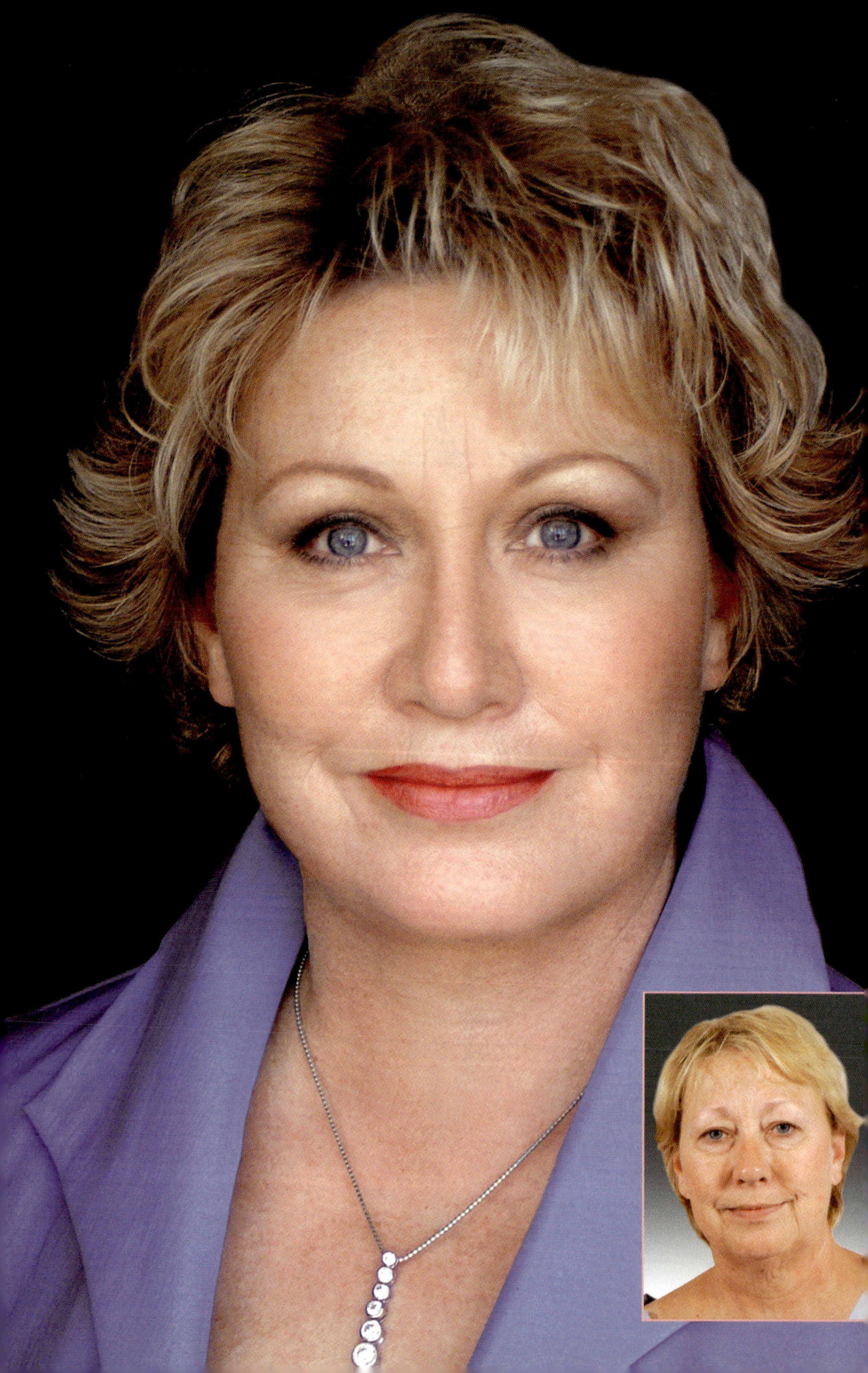

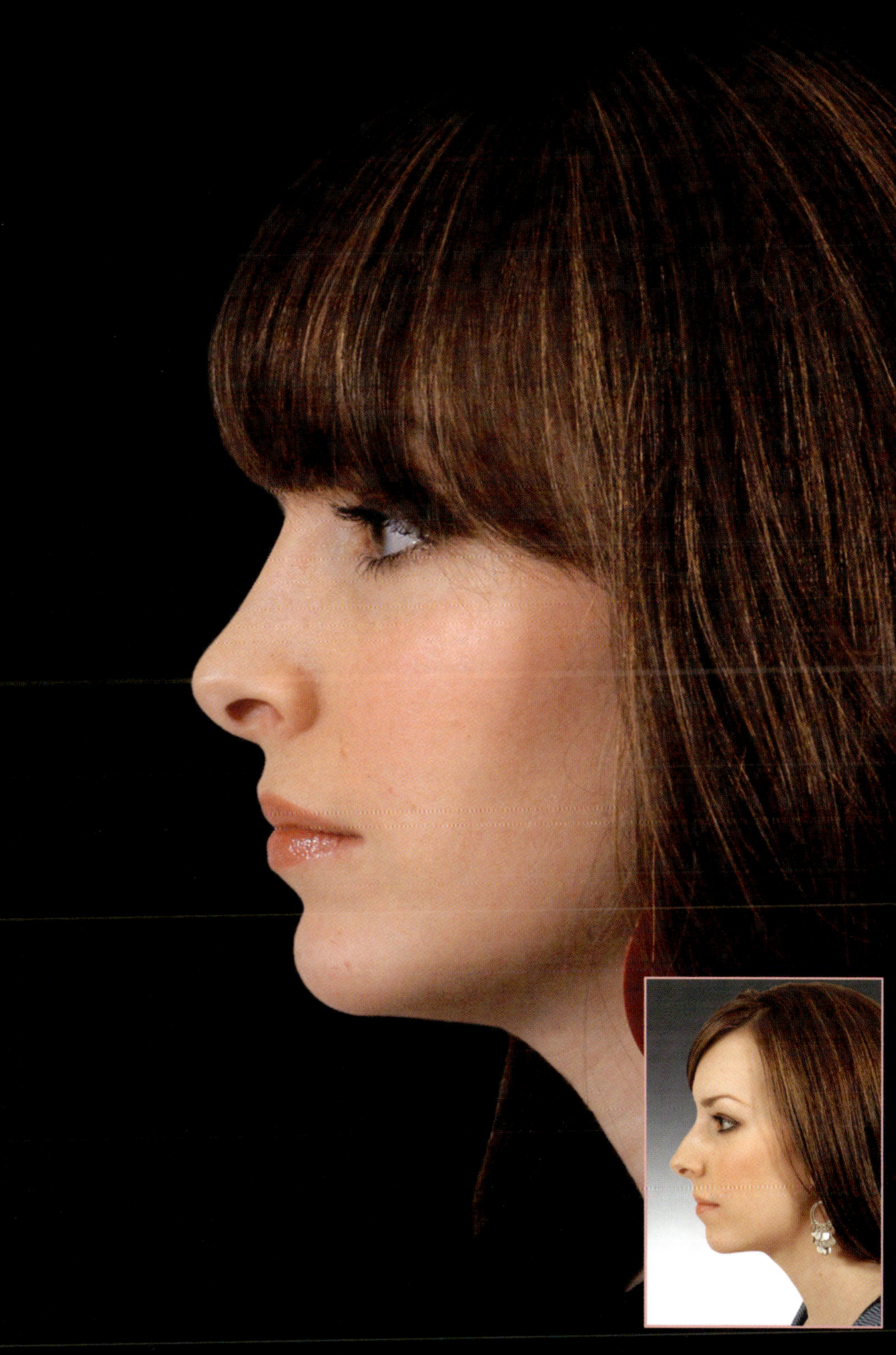

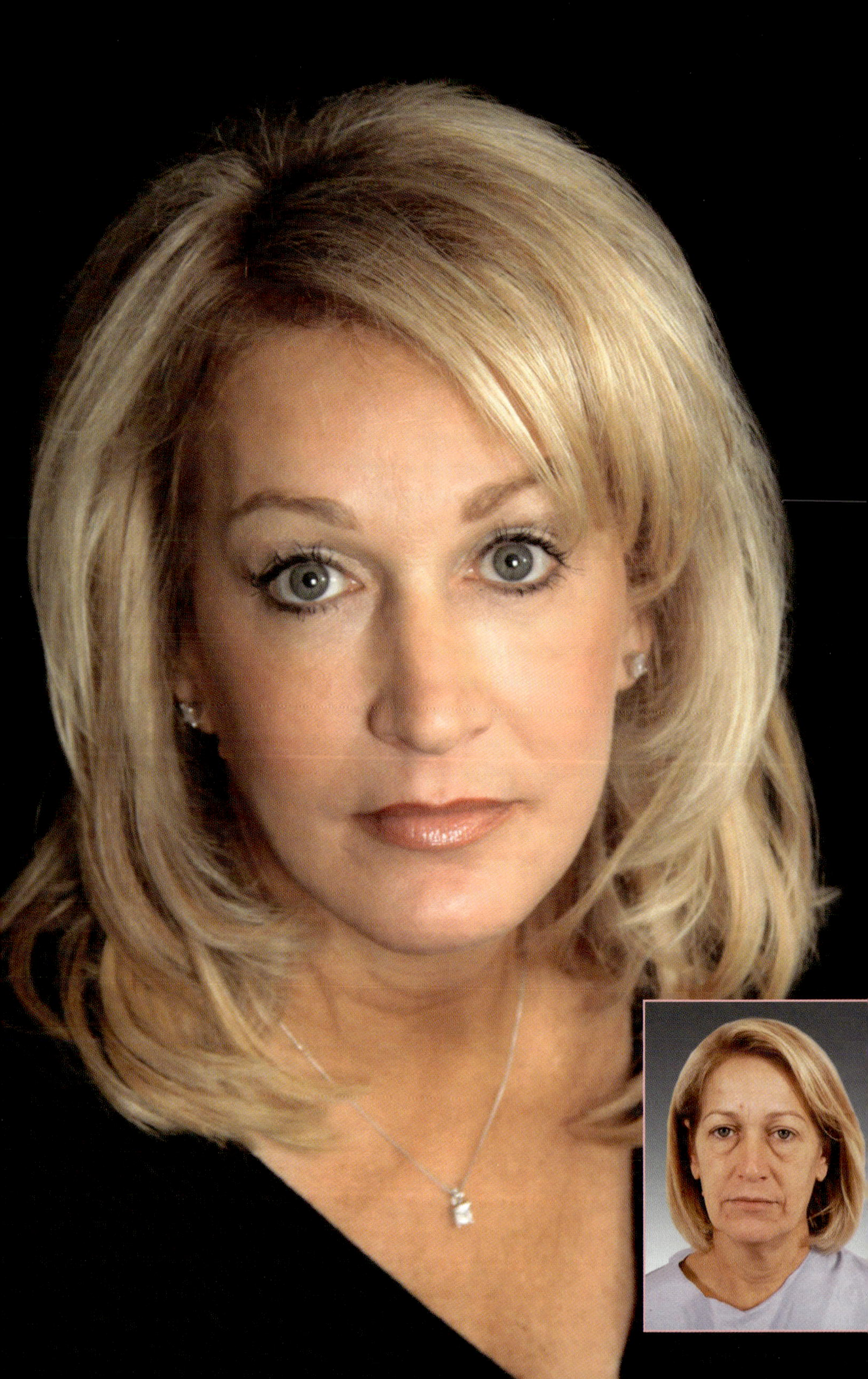

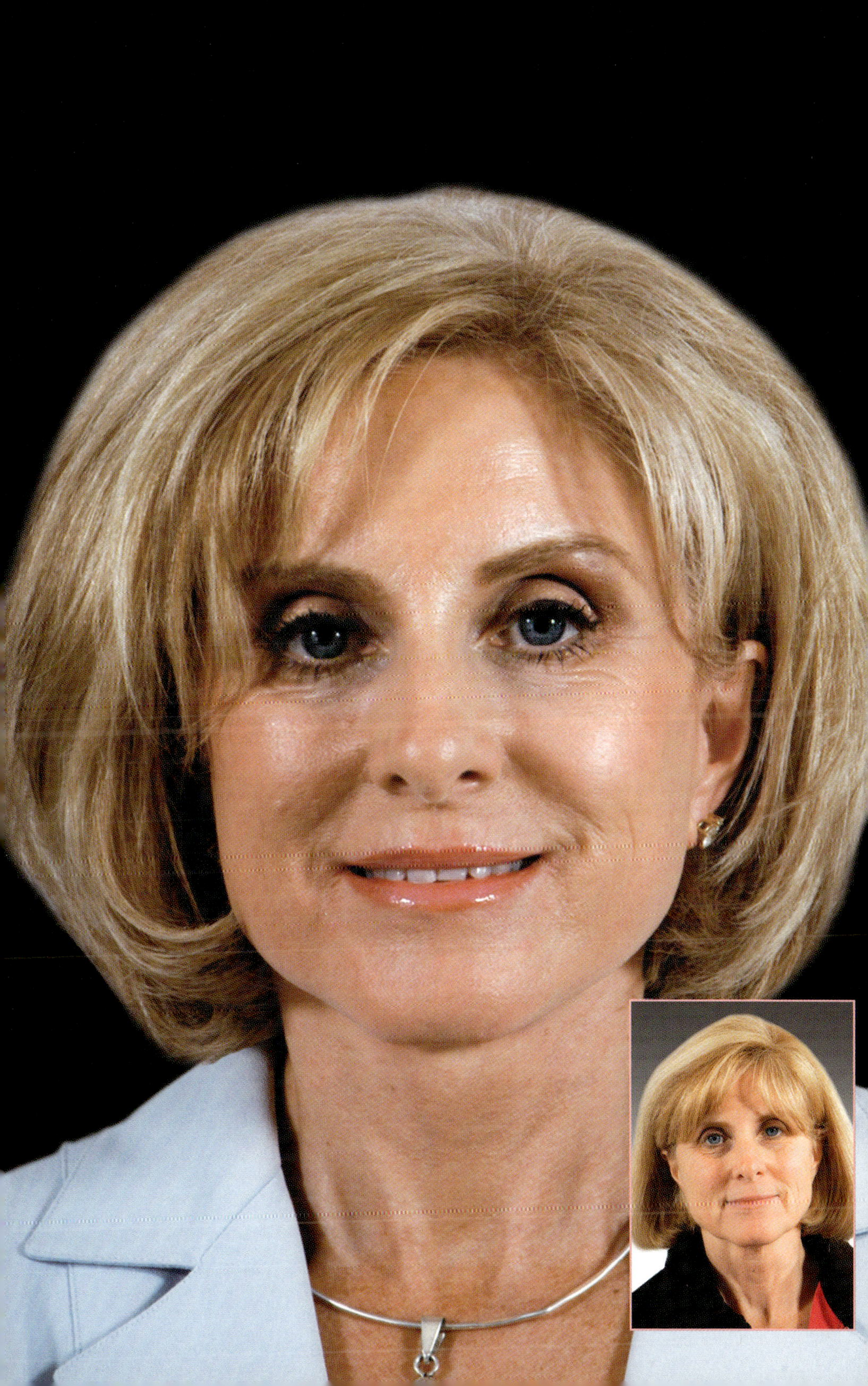

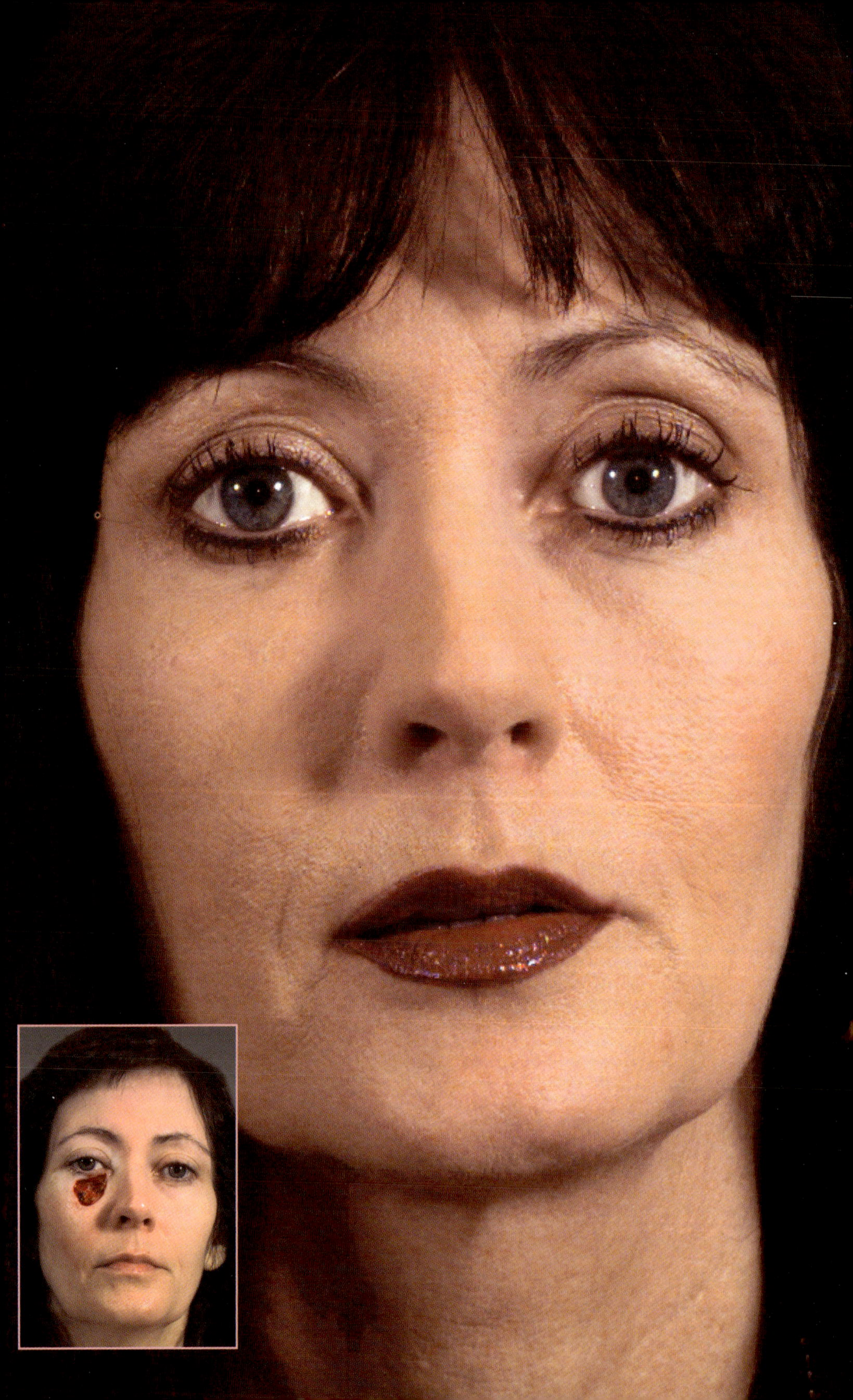

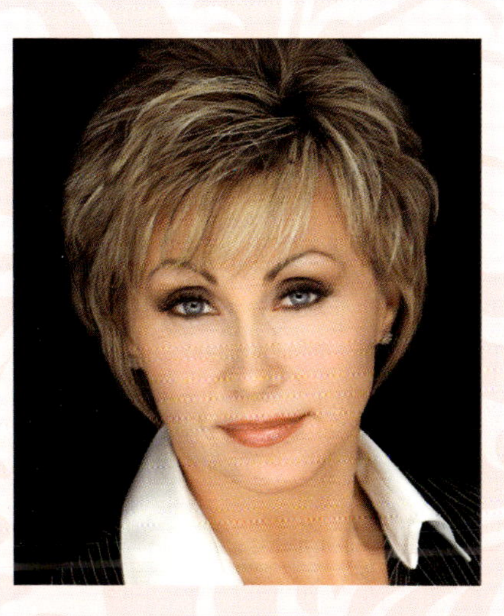

PROCEDURES

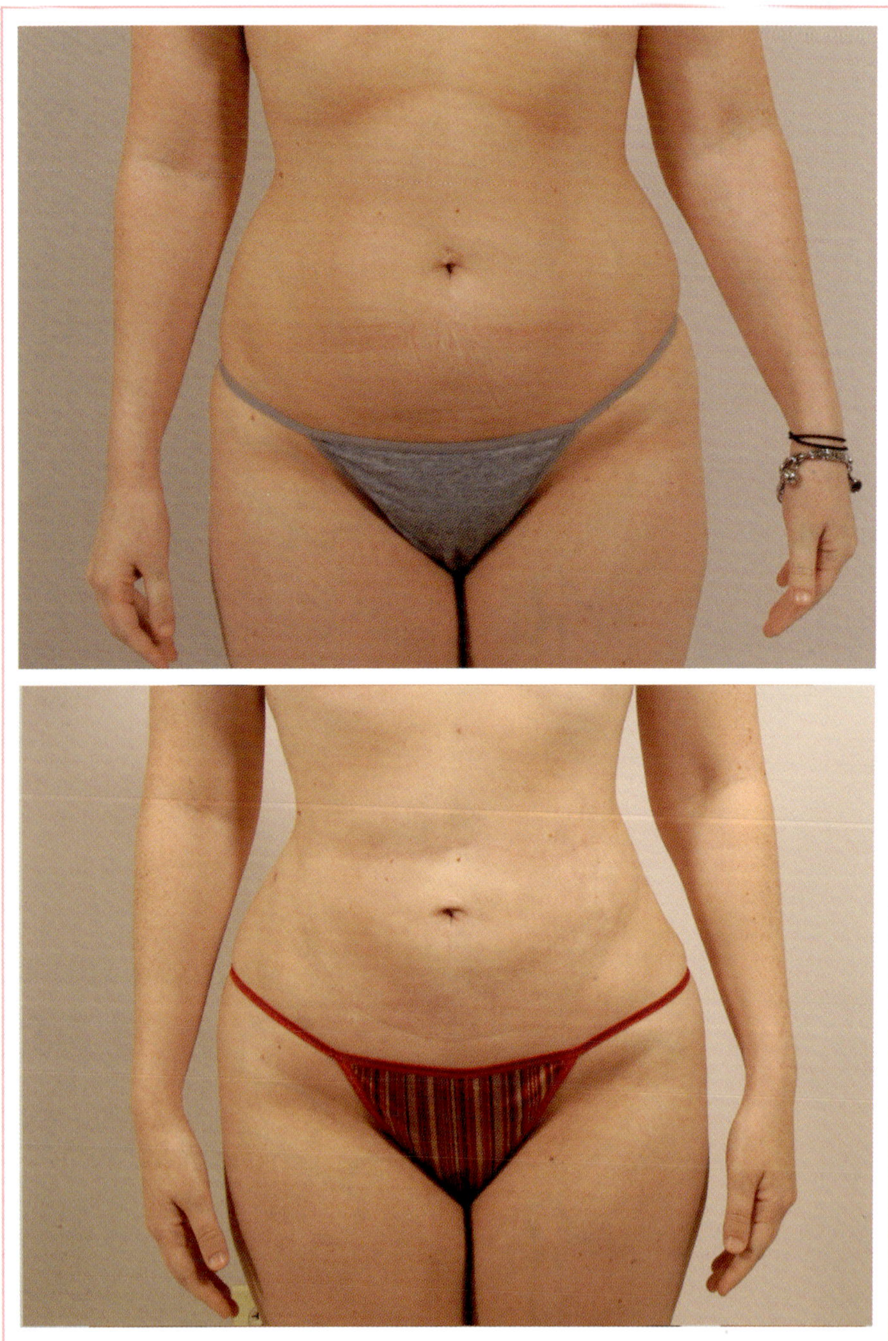

BODY CONTOURING
(Liposuction)

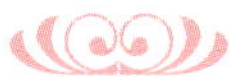

Understanding body contouring

Body contouring, or liposuction, is designed for persons who have specific areas with fat deposits and have tried unsuccessfully to eliminate them through diet, exercise, or weight loss. Body contouring removes fat cells beneath the skin in order to improve the shape of those areas. The procedure can be performed nearly any place on the body, and has proven particularly effective in the abdomen, waist, hips, and thighs. It can also be used on the arms, buttocks, knees and ankles. Body contouring is suitable for both men and women who are in good health.

In consultation, the surgeon considers the objectives of the clients, their problem areas and skin elasticity before making a recommendation for body contouring. The results of body contouring are often remarkable, but it is unrealistic to expect perfection. Clients should presume that the irregularities and dimpling of the skin present before body contouring are likely to remain following the procedure. While improving the overall shape of the body, the procedure usually does not improve cellulite.

The fat that is removed during body contouring cannot return. This is not to say that one cannot gain weight following surgery. A weight gain following this procedure results in a more generalized heaviness with fewer predispositions for fat deposits in the treated areas. Body contouring is usually not an appropriate treatment for obesity and is no substitute for good nutrition and regular exercise. However, obese clients may be suitable candidates for body liposuction if their goal is simply a reduction in body size. In addition, clients must be in good general health and committed to avoid additional weight gain.

Understanding the procedure

Body contouring is performed as an outpatient procedure, usually under general anesthesia. Prior to the procedure, the areas to be treated are carefully marked to guide the surgeon. Cannulas are inserted through very small punctures in the skin to suction out excess fat. Scarring from the procedure usually becomes imperceptible over time.

Improvements in body contouring techniques require the surgeon to inject moderate amounts of fluid into the targeted areas before removing fatty deposits. The fluid contains agents designed to limit blood loss and reduce discomfort. This technique also makes the recovery period much easier. A further innovation in body contouring is the use of very fine cannulas. These cannulas allow the surgeon to use a tiny puncture instead of an incision and to approach fat tissue from many sites and directions. The final result is a smoother surgical outcome with a more rapid recovery.

Understanding the recovery

The patient wears elastic garments after the surgery. These garments are removed the morning after surgery so the patient may shower and wash and dry the garments. After showering, the garments are replaced and worn day and night for the next 48 to 72 hours. Some patients need to wear the garments for four to seven days after the surgery. However, many patients choose to wear them longer because of the comfort they provide.

A large volume of fluid drains from the puncture sites during the first 24 to 48 hours following surgery. In general, if there is more drainage there will be less bruising and swelling. Massaging and/or therapeutic ultrasound treatments after body contouring may be beneficial to the overall outcome.

Certain activities are restricted to aid healing. However, most patients are able to engage in light activity the day after surgery. Normal activity can be resumed within a week or so, but soreness should be expected. Exposure to the sun is to be avoided during healing because it may darken the small, maturing scars.

Once the excess fat is removed, the body takes several months to tighten the loose skin provided the patient's skin has not lost the ability to do so. This process begins in two to four weeks and progresses slowly. The best result from body contouring is achieved in six to twelve months following the procedure and can be greatly enhanced if the patient continues to lose weight through diet and exercise.

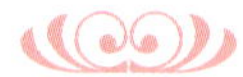

BREAST SURGERY

(Augmentation, Reduction Mammoplasty, Vertical Mammoplasty and Mastopexy)

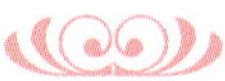

Understanding breast surgery

The goal of breast surgery is to improve the size, shape and appearance of the breasts. Because a woman's body build is primarily determined by genetic and environmental influences, she may not be able to achieve the look she desires through diet and exercise alone. Today, surgical techniques allow a woman to alter the size and shape of her breasts through breast augmentation, breast reduction and/or breast lift. An important part of the preoperative consultation includes a determination of the desired breast size and shape. Although many different breast contours can be achieved, a decision must be made that coincides with total body size, shape and the existing breast tissue.

BREAST AUGMENTATION: Some women with small or asymmetrical breasts choose to undergo breast augmentation. This procedure improves the contour of a woman's body by implanting specially designed saline-filled or silicone implants directly beneath breast tissue or the chest wall muscle. Incision placement varies depending on patient and surgeon preference. Many surgeons prefer to place the implants beneath the chest wall muscle. This placement usually results in softer and more natural looking breasts both standing and lying down. It also may decrease the possibility of unnaturally firm and painful breasts while also improving the reliability of mammograms.

BREAST REDUCTION (Reduction mammoplasty): Women with unusually large, sagging, or uneven breasts may be helped through breast reduction. This surgery reduces the dissatisfaction some women experience due to discomfort that results from the size of their breasts or the pressure of bra straps on their shoulders. Large breasts may also interfere with physical activities and make it difficult to find clothes that fit properly.

The typical breast reduction technique is performed by making an incision around the areola. The incision is extended downward to the base of the breast where it joins with a horizontal incision in the crease. The incision below the areola forms an upside-down T.

Another method of breast reduction is VERTICAL MAMMOPLASTY. This procedure is performed by making an incision that circles the areola and extends down vertically to the base of the breast. The best candidates for this type of breast procedure are 1) women who have breast tissue that has fallen and desire that it be repositioned or 2) women with moderately large breasts that desire a breast reduction and lift. Known as the "lollipop" technique, this procedure allows the surgeon to achieve rounder, fuller breasts with a more desirable shape.

BREAST LIFT (Mastopexy): This procedure repositions or "lifts" breasts that sag as a result of pregnancy and nursing or a large weight gain followed by weight loss. These conditions cause the amount of breast tissue to decrease, leaving a skin envelope that is too large. The remaining breast tissue sags within the larger skin envelope. Breast lift raises and firms the breasts by removing excess skin and tightening the surrounding tissue to reshape and support the new breast contour. However, this procedure only restructures the skin. When more improvement of underlying tissue is indicated, a vertical mammoplasty should be recommended.

Understanding the procedure

Before the surgery, the breasts are carefully marked to indicate where incisions are to be made. The placement of these incisions depends upon the type of breast surgery that is being performed as well as the technique that will achieve the best result. Every effort is made to reduce the length of scars and to make them as inconspicuous as possible. Breast surgery is performed using general anesthesia as an outpatient procedure.

Understanding the recovery

Discomfort following surgery is generally minimal to moderate and is usually controlled with oral medications. Patients undergoing breast surgery may wear a special bra for several weeks and/or limit activities that interfere with the healing process. They should refrain from strenuous exercise for several days to avoid long-term complications. The internal stitches used to close the incisions dissolve in a few weeks.

Swelling and discoloration may occur but usually subside in a few weeks. Areas of numbness, firmness and tenderness around the incisions and under the skin are common. Normal feeling returns several weeks to months after surgery; however, the sensations of the breasts may never be quite the same particularly with large breast reductions. Scars from the incisions, although permanent, fade significantly with time; 18 to 36 months or longer may be required for this fading process to be completed, especially with breast reduction and breast lifting procedures.

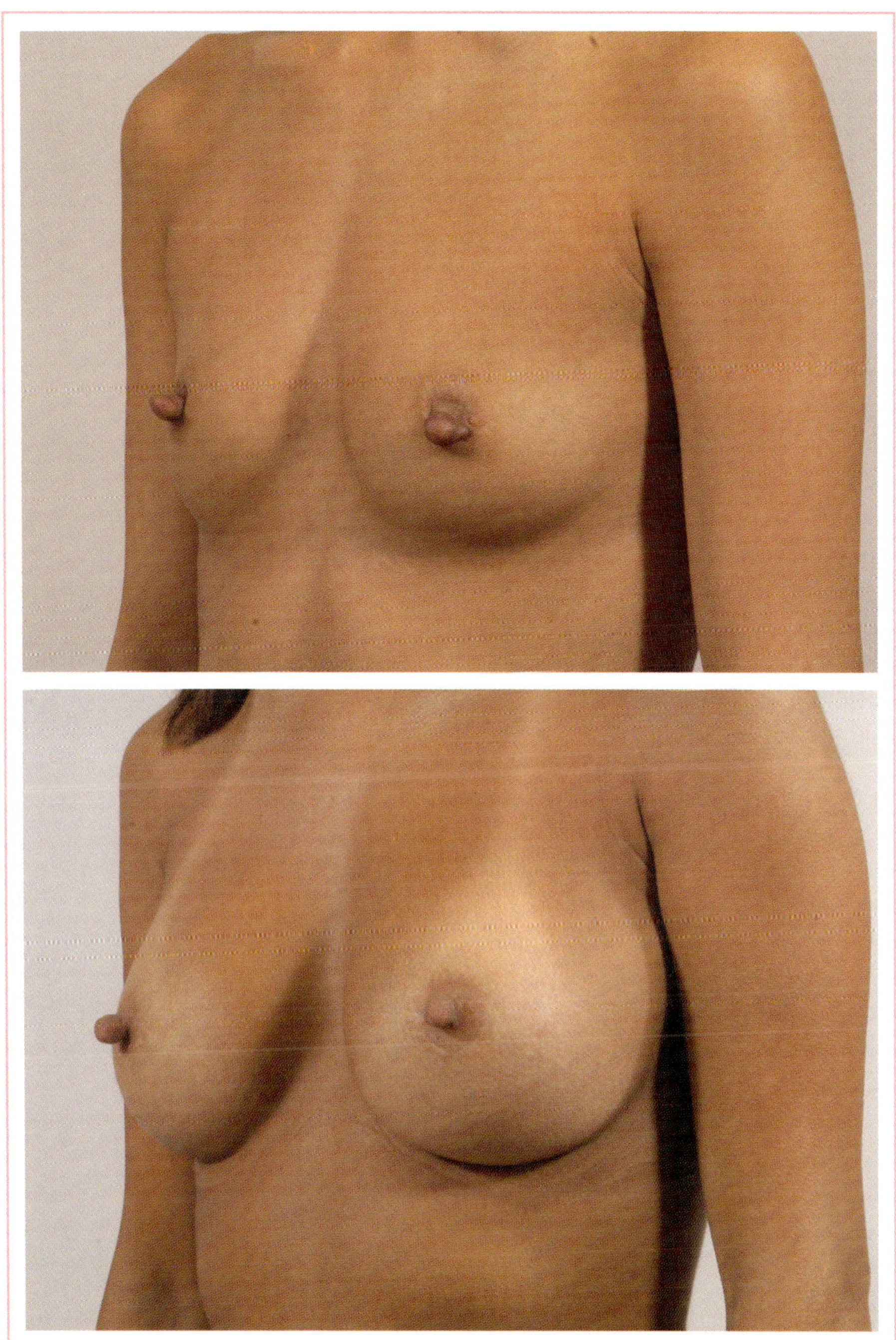

BODY LIFT
(Belt Lipectomy)

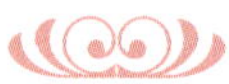

Understanding body lifting

The goal of a body lift, or belt lipectomy, is to remove excess skin and fat in the abdomen, hips, buttocks and thighs. Body lifting involves three procedures performed in one surgical session: tummy tuck, thigh lift and buttock lift. This surgery is commonly performed on individuals who have experienced significant weight loss and have an excess of skin. However, body lifting is also appropriate for patients who desire tightening of the skin to counter the effects of childbearing and aging.

The best candidate for a body lift has had stable weight for a minimum of nine months to a year. He or she should be participating in a regular exercise program and eating a healthy diet. Persons who have had bariatric procedures should wait at least a year after the surgery to allow any health problems associated with obesity to improve. Women who plan future pregnancies may be advised to postpone the procedure until after childbearing.

Understanding the procedure

Surgery is performed under general anesthesia. The time required for the procedure ranges from three to five hours. Although the steps of the body lift differ based on the needs of the patient, the surgeon usually operates on the abdomen first. A horizontal incision is made along the pubic area to remove excess fat and skin. In cases that require the removal of fat, liposuction is performed prior to removing excess skin. Any repairs to the abdominal wall (such as hernia) can be made at this time. In most cases, the belly button is repositioned because of the amount of skin that is removed. The remaining abdominal tissue is pulled down and sutured at the pubic area. The removal of excess fat and skin is then repeated in the buttock and thigh areas.

Although hidden by clothing, a scar is unavoidable. The scar may widen and require surgical improvement at a later time. However, scar revision surgery is uncommon. Every effort is made to minimize the size of the scar and make it as inconspicuous as possible through such methods as taping the incision post-operatively. In spite of the scar, most patients are enthusiastic about their results.

Understanding the recovery

Because body lifting is a major surgical procedure, it requires significant recovery time. Most patients remain in the hospital for one night. Discomfort following surgery is first managed with IV medication and then by oral medicines.

Drainage tubes require personal home care for up to four days. A compression garment is worn at all times except while showering for at least two to six days. Dressings are usually removed two days following surgery.

Following the surgery, there are restrictions on activities such as exercise and lifting. Most people require four to six weeks' recovery before returning to normal activities, and generally from six to eight weeks before exercising. Patients may resume work with some restrictions after three weeks.

Some individuals experience reduced sensation in the treated areas, which can be permanent. The abdominal scars may appear to worsen during the first weeks or months, and may take up to six to nine before they flatten and lighten in color. The final result of this surgery is usually achieved six months to a year after the procedure.

BUTT IMPLANTS
(Buttock Augmentation)

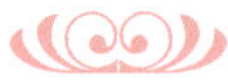

Understanding buttock augmentation

Buttock augmentation (or butt implants) involves the surgical insertion of silicone implants into the buttock area. People who are unhappy with the size or contour of their buttocks request this surgery. Some individuals feel their buttocks lack shape, while others want to appear more full and rounded. Slender women often request implants because their bodies do not have the fat cells needed to create the look they desire through fat transfer.

Often, when women have breast lifts and/or augmentations, the overall proportion of the body is not considered. There are curves in the breast and thigh areas but the buttocks may be flat or poorly shaped. The upper and outer parts of the buttocks can be improved by placing implants on top of or beneath the muscle. To improve the lower area of the buttocks, the implants must be placed on top of the muscle to avoid pressure on the sciatic nerve.

An important part of the preoperative consultation includes discussion of the desired shape and size of the buttocks. This discussion enables Dr. English to determine which size implants will achieve the preferred size and contour. The surgeon also explains the options available including incision type, location of the implant, type of implant, and whether buttocks lifting might also be beneficial.

While buttock augmentation may be indicated as a solitary procedure, it can be combined with other cosmetic procedures such as liposuction and fat transfer to enhance the overall outcome.

Understanding the procedure

Buttock augmentation is performed under general anesthesia as an outpatient procedure. An incision is made in the crease between the buttocks cheeks where the scar will be less noticeable. Dr. English creates a pocket within the tissue of the buttock and inserts the implant either under or on top of the gluteus maximus muscle. The same procedure is performed on the other side; then the surgeon ensures that the buttocks are symmetrical and natural looking. Buttock implant surgery

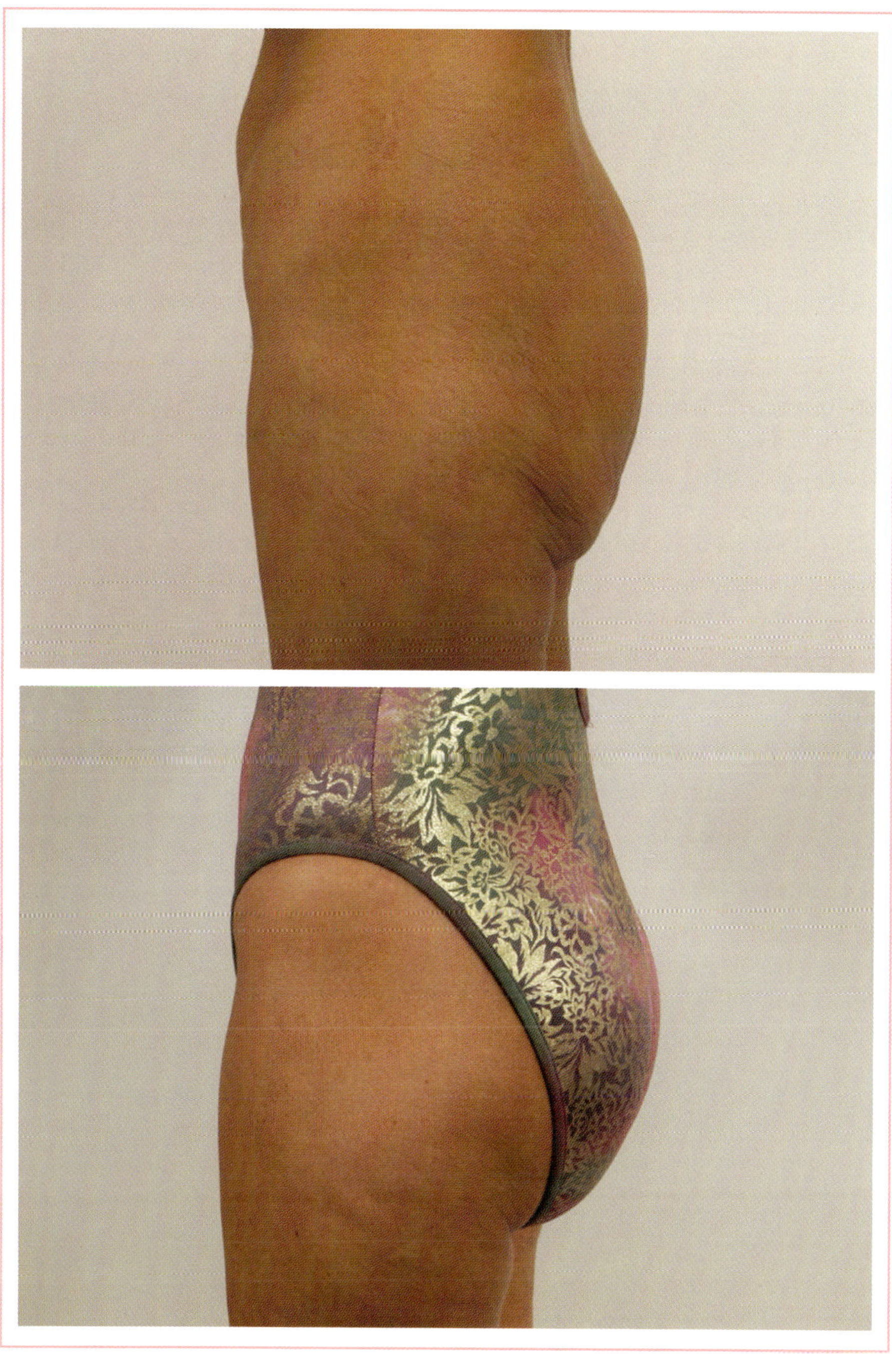

usually takes about two hours depending on the placement of the implants and the patient's anatomy.

Understanding the recovery

Buttock augmentation stretches the tissues and can be painful, especially when the implants are placed within the muscle. Mechanically speaking, the buttocks are one of the most used parts of the body which leads to the discomfort following this procedure. The discomfort is greatest within the first 48 hours, but improves daily and is managed by oral medications.

To provide support, the patient may wear a compression garment day and night until instructed otherwise. The stitches are removed within a week to ten days, but swelling may continue until it gradually subsides over several weeks. As the swelling subsides, the results become more apparent.

Bruising may occur in the surgical area following the procedure. If bruising develops, it should be much improved in two to four weeks. Areas of numbness, firmness and tenderness around the incision and under the skin are common. Normal feeling should return several weeks to months after surgery.

The incision for buttock augmentation carries a significant infection risk. In order to minimize this risk, personal hygiene is of paramount importance. Following the butt implant procedure, the patient should not sit directly on the buttocks for up to three weeks. It is important that the patient avoids resting and sleeping on her back to prevent the implants from shifting.

Most patients are able to resume calm, quiet activities within a few days following the surgery. Physical activity should be avoided for several weeks. Most patients return to work in two weeks provided they do a minimum amount of sitting. Most normal activities can be resumed after four weeks, when the soreness has subsided. However, recovery varies from patient to patient and depends upon the technique, type of implant and site of placement as well as the level of activities in the daily routine.

Since nothing heals symmetrically or suddenly, the best result will usually be achieved in four to six months. In spite of the initial discomfort, most patients are very satisfied with their result.

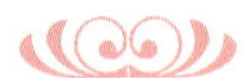

CHEEK IMPLANTS
(Cheek Augmentation)

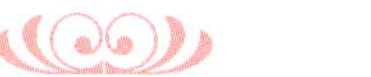

Understanding cheek implants

Cheek implants enhance the cheekbones and/or midface that provides an appearance of elegance and youth. They can give a relatively flat mid face a more attractive contour. They often add a finishing touch and provide balance for those seeking better facial harmony. Although most patients who elect to have cheek implant surgery are women, many men choose this surgery.

Recent improvements in surgical materials have resulted in a variety of sizes and shapes of implants. The implants are carefully designed to fit the skeletal form resulting in a very natural appearance. All implants are composed of materials that have been found safe following many years of surgical use.

During the initial consultation, the surgeon analyzes the face and discusses the patient's objectives. If surgery is indicated, the appropriate implant for each patient and for each cheek is selected. When the face is asymmetrical prior to surgery, some asymmetry may be present following the procedure.

While cheek implant surgery may be indicated as a solitary procedure, it is commonly combined with other cosmetic procedures to enhance the overall outcome. Cheek implant surgery is frequently performed with facelift, eyelid surgery and/or nose surgery to achieve an optimum result.

Understanding the procedure

Immediately following the surgery, the surgeon may apply a pressure bandage that is removed in the office the next day.

Cheek implant surgery is usually performed using local anesthesia with I.V. sedation as an outpatient procedure. Depending on the patient's profile, the implants are inserted at or below the natural cheekbone by creating a small tunnel underneath the upper lip via an intraoral incision. The incision is closed with absorbable sutures to avoid the need for removal. The procedure heals with no external scarring.

Understanding the recovery

Recovery is rapid although there may be mild to moderate discomfort that is controlled with oral medications. Chewing is limited immediately after cheek implant surgery and a liquid or soft food diet is required for several days. Some activities such as heavy lifting and bending are limited for several days following the procedure. Facial expressions and movements are also restricted to prevent the implant from shifting. Pressure to the cheek areas should be avoided for four to six weeks.

Although the cheek areas are swollen initially and some bruising may occur, most of the swelling subsides in a few days. Numb and firm areas around the cheeks and mouth are common, but are self-limiting. Most patients return to work or resume normal activities within a few days after surgery.

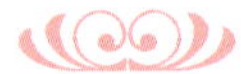

CHIN IMPLANT
(Mentoplasty)

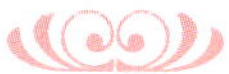

Understanding chin implants

Chin implantation creates a pleasing balanced profile by inserting a medical-grade implant to build up a recessed chin. This device is frequently used to improve a "weak" chin that may be the result of development, trauma or heredity. Chin implant improves facial harmony and often results in increased self-confidence. It is one of the more gratifying procedures in facial profile correction. The improvement can be dramatic.

Recent improvements in surgical materials have resulted in implants that become minimally incorporated into the chin tissue to prevent potential shifting. Implants are available in many shapes and sizes so the procedure can be customized for each patient. Shortly after implantation, the materials become attached to the surrounding tissue. Materials that compose the implants have been used for many years and are considered safe.

During consultation, the surgeon analyzes the chin and jaw to determine if an implant will improve the facial profile. In considering the profile, the chin projection should usually be even with or slightly in front of a vertical line drawn downward from the lower lip. A well-defined chin gives balance to the face and creates a major portion of the profile.

Many surgeons recommend a chin implant along with nose surgery, a face lift or facial liposuction. This recommendation is made because the surgeon does not consider the chin as an isolated structure, but as an important feature of the face. The combination of procedures may result in better facial harmony.

Understanding the procedure

A chin implantation is performed using local anesthesia with I.V. sedation as an outpatient procedure. A small incision is made either in the natural crease line just under the chin or inside the mouth just above where the gum and lower lip meet. The implant is inserted into a small space that is created by Dr. English and fine sutures are used to close the incision. If the incision is inside the mouth, no external scarring

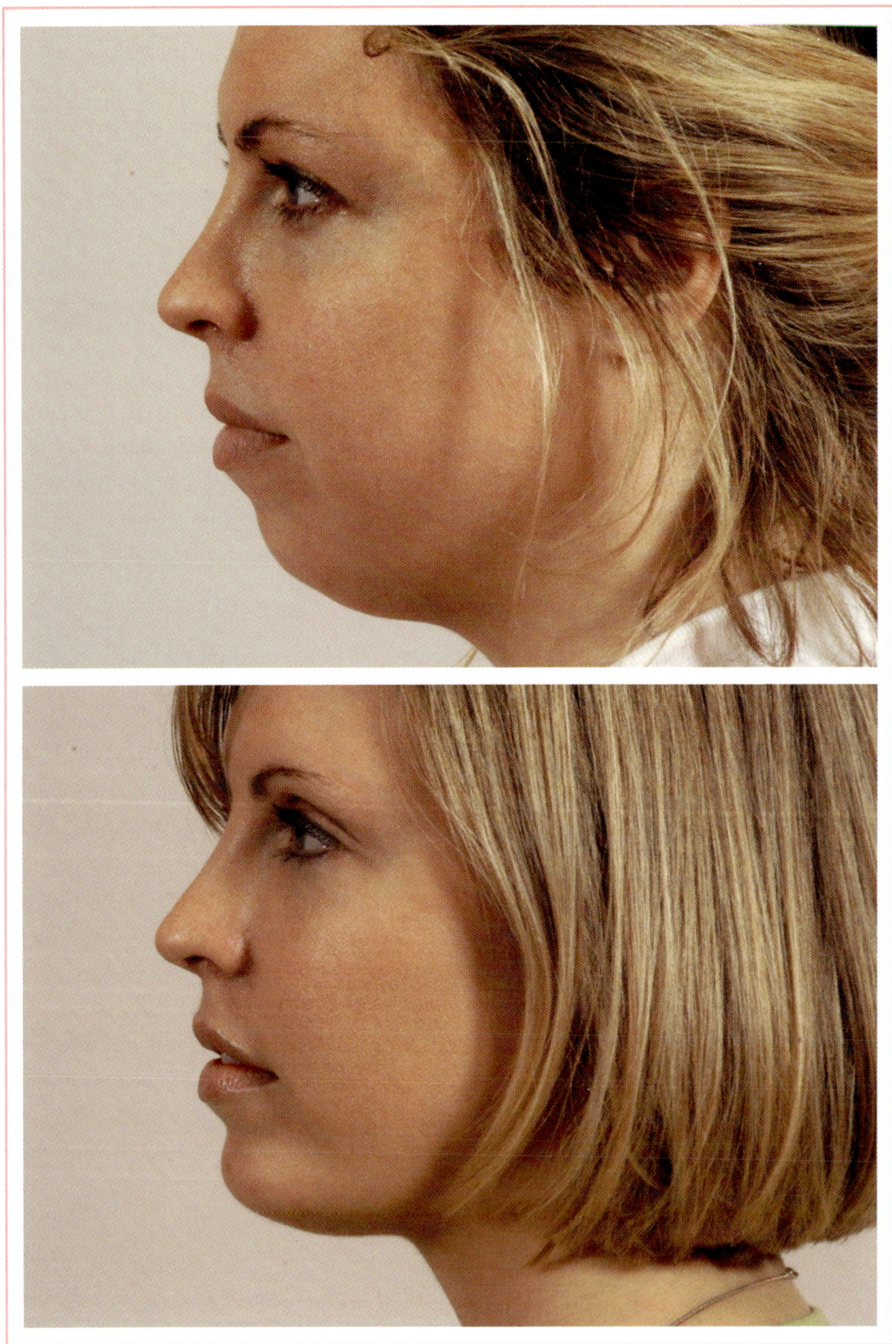

is visible. If the incision is under the chin, the scar fades over time, becoming nearly imperceptible.

Understanding the recovery

Immediately after the procedure, Dr. English may apply a pressure bandage that is removed in the office the day after the surgery. After the pressure bandage is removed, there may be tape over the incision. This tape stays in place for five to seven days and is removed at the next office visit.

Recovery is rapid although there is mild to moderate discomfort that is controlled with oral medications. Chewing is limited immediately after chin surgery and a liquid or soft food diet is required for a few days if the incision is in the mouth. Some activities, such as heavy lifting and bending, are limited for several days following the procedure. Facial expressions are also restricted for two to four weeks to prevent the implant from shifting.

Numb and firm areas are somewhat common following chin surgery but are rarely long lasting. After approximately three to twelve weeks, most of the numbness as well as the swelling and bruising are gone. The inconvenience of this procedure is rarely an issue with patients who need this type of profile correction.

EYELID SURGERY
(Blepharoplasty)

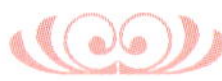

Understanding eyelid surgery

Eyelid surgery, or blepharoplasty, is chosen by many men and women to correct bags and bulges around the eyes as well as drooping eyelids. Although more women than men choose eyelid surgery, the procedure is equally suited for both genders.

People of all ages have eyelid surgery. Younger patients have the surgery because of an inherited condition in which fat cushions of the eye push forward causing a bulging appearance. Older patients generally have eyelid surgery to reduce these bulges as well as the sagging of eyelid skin. Droopy eyelids can make a person look older and in some cases, impair vision. Eyelid surgery results in a refreshed appearance with a more youthful eye area.

During a consultation, Dr. English asks about vision, tear production, use of contact lenses and expectations. This information plus age, skin type, ethnic background and degree of visual obstruction is assessed to determine the best course of treatment. Eyelid surgery does not normally reduce wrinkling around the eye area nor does it lift a drooping brow. Therefore, many patients decide to combine eyelid surgery with other procedures such as a forehead and brow lift, fat transfer, mid facelift or skin resurfacing to achieve the best overall result.

Understanding the procedure

Eyelid surgery is performed in the office with local anesthesia under I.V. sedation. The procedure normally takes less than one hour. Upper and lower eyelid surgery may be performed at the same time; however, either can be done independently.

Upper eyelid surgery is performed by making an incision in the natural crease of the eyelid. Excess skin and fat are removed through the incision, which is closed with fine sutures, thereby minimizing the visibility of any scar.

In lower eyelid surgery, the incision is made in an inconspicuous site along the lash line and smile creases of the lower lid or more commonly on the inside of the eyelid. Once excess tissue, skin and/or fat is removed, absorbable sutures are used to

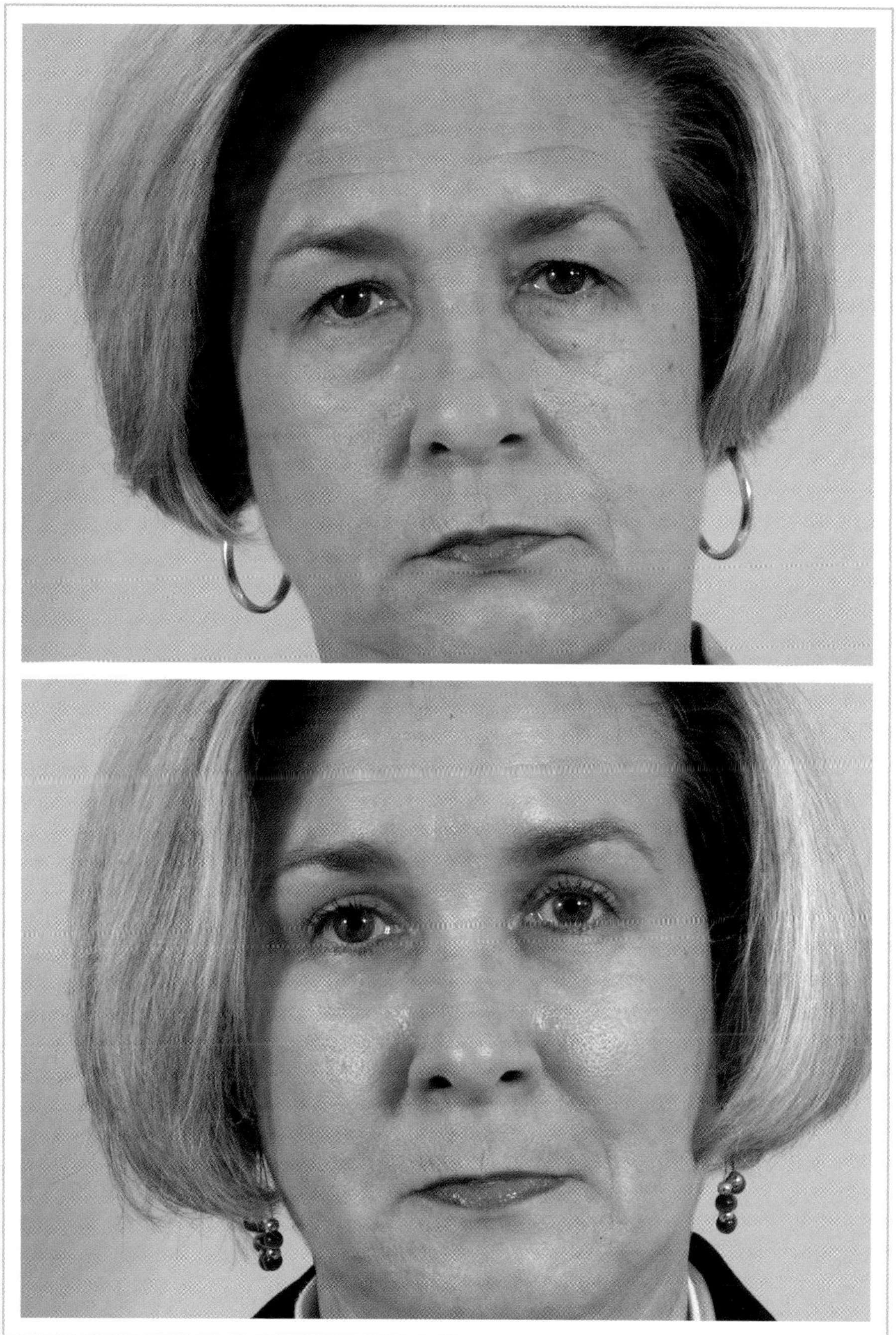

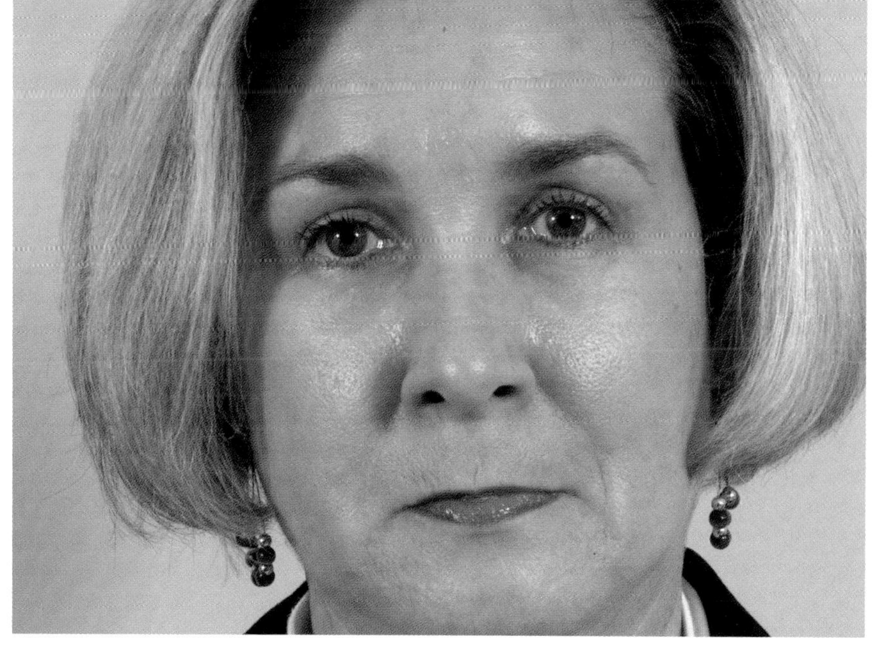

close the incisions. This technique is increasingly chosen, especially when performed along with a chemical peel and/or laser resurfacing. Eyelid puffiness of the lower lid that is caused only by excess fat is corrected by removing excess fatty tissue through an incision made inside the eyelid. No visible scar results from this type of procedure.

Understanding the recovery

Most patients experience little or no discomfort following eyelid surgery and find that any discomfort is relieved by taking a mild analgesic. Following surgery, patients are instructed on cleaning the incisions and the application of antibiotic eye ointment when indicated.

Some swelling and bruising may develop after the procedure. Cold compresses, as well as head elevation enhances healing and relieves discomfort. As time passes, the incisions for both the upper and lower eyelids blend in with the surrounding skin and are easily camouflaged. The skin at the outer corners of the eye is thicker and takes a bit longer to heal.

The stitches used to close the incisions in the upper and lower eyelids are removed five to six days after surgery. The sun may darken maturing scars; therefore, incisions in the upper and lower eyelids should be protected by sunscreen, sunglasses, or a hat as they heal.

Most patients can return to near normal activity within a few days of the surgery. However, as the incisions heal, it is important to restrict activities that may put pressure on the eyes. Lifting, bending, and straining should be avoided for up to two weeks. Aerobic or heavy exercise should be avoided for at least three weeks following surgery.

Most patients can anticipate a marked improvement in the appearance of their eyes. This is often accompanied by a feeling of tightness in the eyelids that may last a few weeks. Bags and bulges are significantly reduced if not completely eliminated. Some patients may actually experience slight improvement in their eyesight or peripheral vision as a result of the removal of excess skin.

For those patients with a sunken look to their lower eyelid area, fat transfer to these areas combined with a chemical peel can help restore a more youthful contour from lash to cheek area. Normally, the reason for this loss of volume is due to the descent of cheek tissue away from the rim of the eye socket. This type of restoration has been extremely popular during the past decade because it is a relatively minor but extremely successful procedure.

FACELIFT
(Rhytidectomy)

Understanding facelift

The goal of a facelift, or rhytidectomy, is to reduce sagging and loose skin in the face and neck by lifting or repositioning the skin and underlying tissues. As a result of recent improvements in procedures, the facelift has become one of the most desired cosmetic surgeries.

As individuals age, the skin as well as the fat and bone structure of the face change. These changes combine with lifelong facial muscle activity and gravity to create more prominent skin folds, particularly under the chin, in the upper neck and lower facial areas. Face lifting is designed to improve these facial changes. Modern techniques tighten the deeper layers of facial tissue more than the skin and yield a more natural look that may "subtract" eight to twelve years from an individual's appearance. Many patients experience increased self-confidence as a result of having a facelift.

As in all cosmetic surgery, good health and realistic expectations are essential. There is no "ideal" facelift. The surgeon must consider skin type, medical history, skin elasticity, and bone structure among other things in personalizing this procedure. Communication between the patient and the surgeon is essential in obtaining a realistic and positive outcome.

In order to achieve the most desirable effect, many patients decide to combine several cosmetic procedures. Eyelid surgery, facial liposuction, a forehead or brow lift and skin resurfacing are often performed along with a facelift. Combining procedures may be necessary to achieve the best overall result.

Understanding the procedure

Some surgeons prefer to perform a facelift in their office or as an outpatient at a surgery center. The procedure can be performed by using local anesthesia with deep I.V. sedation or general anesthesia. The surgery normally takes two to three hours. Medications are given before surgery to reduce anxiety and stress. Most patients have little or no memories after the preoperative medication is given and regain full awareness in the recovery room or after they have returned home. A turban-type dressing is placed around the head after surgery and is removed in the office the following

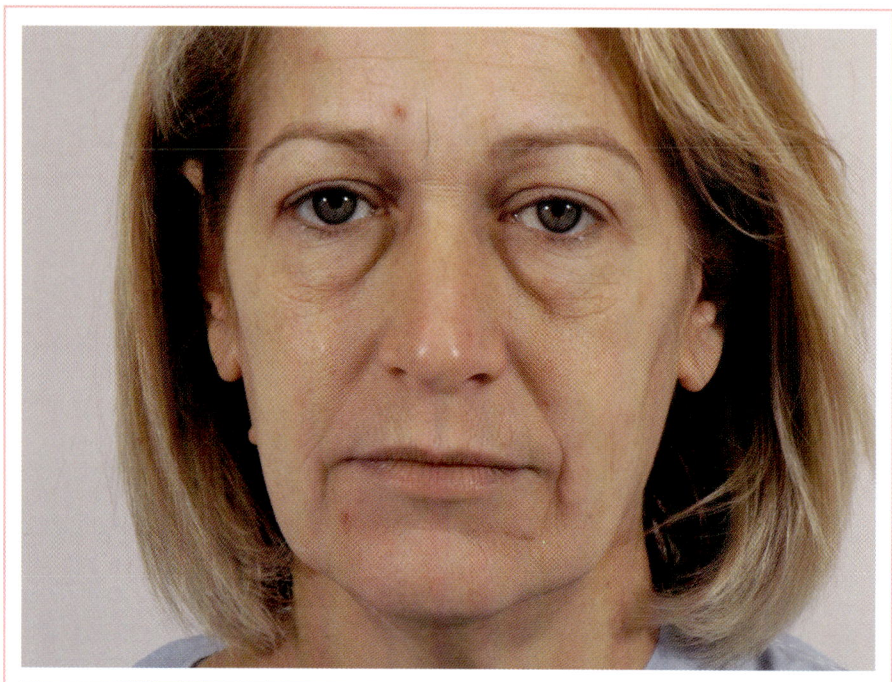

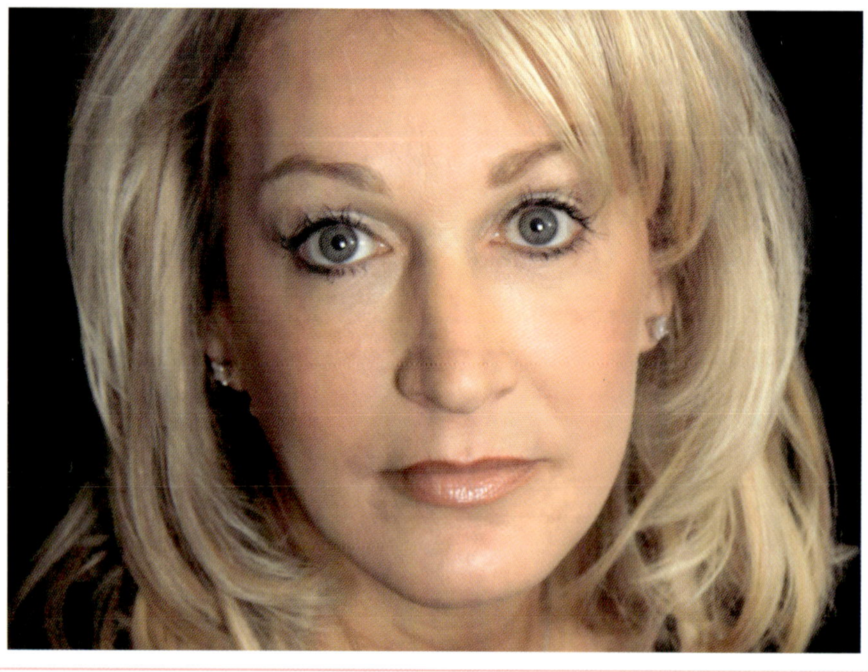

morning. The discomfort following a facelift is usually mild to moderate. Medications are prescribed to help the patient rest comfortably for the first few days after surgery.

The placement of incisions for a facelift varies depending on the problems to be corrected. Consideration is also given to whether the patient is male or female and their respective hair patterns. In all cases, most of the incisions are placed in areas where they will be hidden by hair or natural skin folds. In exposed areas, very fine absorbable sutures are used to close the incisions so the scars should become practically imperceptible over time. Removal of stitches and staples occurs within one week following surgery and causes little discomfort.

Understanding the recovery

Swelling of the face and neck peak at 72 hours. Resting and sleeping in an elevated position helps to reduce swelling and increase the patient's comfort. As a general rule, 80% of the swelling resolves in two to three weeks. The remainder usually subsides over the next two to four months. Bruising may occur in the face and neck and, if it develops, is usually gone in three to six weeks. Areas of numbness, firmness and tenderness around the incisions are common. Normal feeling should return several weeks to months after surgery.

Certain activities are restricted after a facelift to protect healing tissues. Movements such as coughing, sneezing, bending, turning or twisting the head or any exercise are limited for a minimum of three to six weeks. Driving, which often involves twisting the head and neck, can be resumed after two to three weeks. Contact sports are not recommended for at least three to four months. The patient must wait at least 6 weeks to have hair permed or colored.

Since nothing heals symmetrically or suddenly, the best results are achieved three to six months after surgery. The best outcome is achieved by communicating with Dr. English and meticulously following instructions.

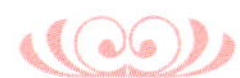

FAT TRANSFER
(Autologous Fat Transplantation or Micro-Lipoinjection)

Understanding fat transfer

Fat transfer involves removing body fat from one location and moving it to another. The goal of the procedure is to improve contour, correct defects or enhance features. For example, fat can be transferred from the abdomen to replace facial fat that is lost due to aging, to enlarge lips or to augment the buttocks (also called "Brazilian butt lift"). Transferred fat lasts longer in areas of non-movement. So the procedure is very successful for the correction of facial hollows and aging of the hands. But not every area of the body is appropriate for fat transfer. In some instances, the breasts should not be injected because fat may reduce the accuracy of mammograms.

Fat injections are semi-permanent and a variable amount of any injected fat will not survive the transfer process. It is not uncommon to require a repeat of fat injections to maintain the final desirable result. Occasionally, no matter how many times fat is injected, it will not "take" or stay in a particular area. However, because fat transfer uses an individual's own fat cells, it cannot be rejected or cause an allergic reaction.

Understanding the procedure

Fat transfer is performed as an outpatient procedure. Using a small cannula attached to a syringe, fat is removed from a donor site where the fat is most tightly packed, such as the hips, abdomen or buttocks.

Once removed, the fat is processed to remove excess fluids and placed into smaller syringes for injection. The transferred fat is injected into the treatment site under the skin and/or deeper into the tissue. This process may be repeated until the desired result has been achieved. The one or two tiny punctures made to remove and inject the fat require no sutures. Although fat transfer can be performed as a solitary procedure, it is frequently performed with facelift, liposuction and eyelid surgery in order to achieve the best result.

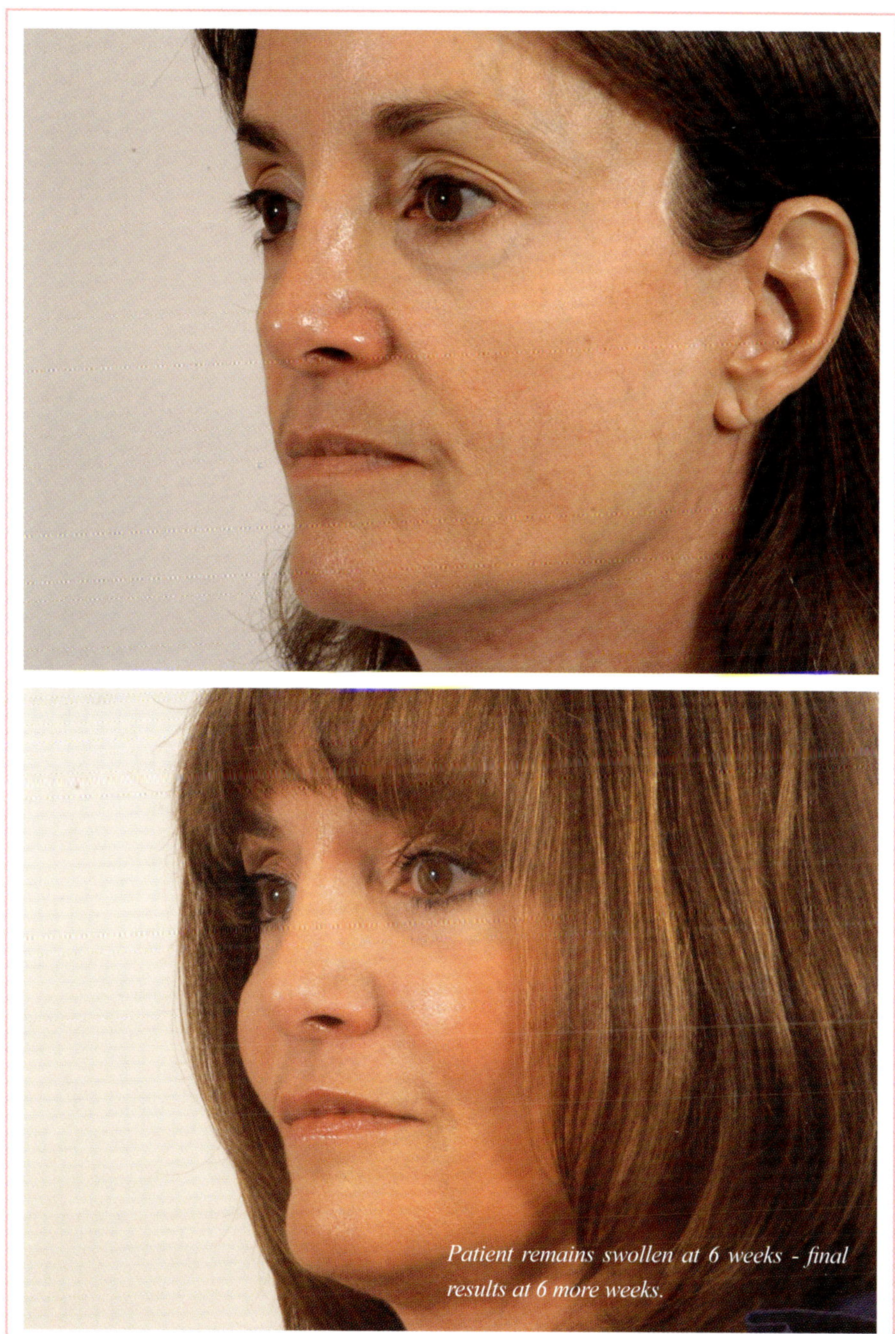
Patient remains swollen at 6 weeks - final
results at 6 more weeks.

Understanding the recovery

The recovery time from fat transfer is almost negligible. Discomfort following the procedure is usually mild and is controlled with medication. In most cases, patients return to normal activities almost immediately. Bruising, swelling and tightness are common and resolve in a few days and/or weeks. Complications, while rare, include infection and areas of reduced sensation which is usually temporary.

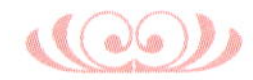

FOREHEAD LIFT and BROW LIFT
(and Endoscopic Laser Forehead Lift)

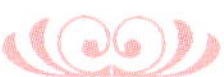

Understanding forehead and brow lift surgery

A forehead lift brow lift, or endoscopic forehead lift moves the eyebrows and adjacent structures back to where they belong, at or above the brow bone. These procedures may also smooth the furrows in the lower mid forehead as well as reduce the drooping skin above the eyes. As a result of the surgery, the eyes appear more open, rested and youthful.

Drooping eyebrows are often one of the first signs of aging. This condition is frequently overlooked because most people are unaware of the problem and the amount of improvement correction can provide. Drooping brows can cause the upper eyelids to sag. In extreme cases, the eyelid skin can touch or overlap the eyelashes. People often comment that their eyes appear to be getting smaller or more deeply set. A drooping brow contributes to the tired look observed at the end of the day. This condition frequently causes eye makeup to end up on the upper part of the eyelids soon after it is applied.

Forehead lift, brow lift or endoscopic forehead lift surgery lessens hooding and the deeper "crow's feet" next to the outer corners of the eye. But it does not reduce lines around the eyes. Also, the lift does not correct excess skin or fat deposits in the lids. In order to achieve the best result, Dr. English may recommend combining forehead lift, brow lift or endoscopic forehead lift with other procedures such as eyelid surgery, facelift or Botulinum toxin injections.

Understanding the procedure

During consultation, the surgeon analyzes the eyes, brows, forehead and hairline to determine the placement of the incisions. In forehead lift surgery, incisions are usually placed behind the hairline of the scalp or at the hairline where the forehead and scalp meet. Placement depends upon the height of the patient's hairline. In order to achieve a natural result, it is critical to avoid appreciably altering the hair pattern. The incisions for a brow lift are placed on the forehead or above the brows only when especially indicated. Incisions for endoscopic forehead lift are made above or at the hairline. In any case, great care is taken to place incisions within the hair, hairline, or naturally occurring folds of skin to make the resulting scars as inconspicuous as possible.

Forehead lift, brow lift and endoscopic forehead lift surgeries are outpatient procedures performed under local anesthesia with I. V. sedation or general anesthesia. A turban-type head dressing may be placed following surgery and is removed in the office the following day. The discomfort following a forehead, brow lift or endoscopic forehead lift is usually minimal to moderate. Oral medications help the patient rest comfortably after surgery. Removal of the stitches and/or staples occurs after five to six days and creates little discomfort.

Understanding the recovery

Swelling of the forehead peaks around 72 hours and as a general rule is not noticeable after one to two weeks. Resting and sleeping in an elevated position helps to reduce swelling and increase comfort. Bruising rarely occurs in the forehead but may appear under the eyes. If bruising develops, it is gone in three to six weeks. Most patients experience itching sensations during the healing process. Areas of numbness, firmness and tenderness around the incisions are common. Normal sensations gradually return within several weeks to months after the surgery. Although an uncommon effect, scalp sensation may never be quite the same.

Certain activities are restricted after a forehead or brow lift to protect healing tissues. Facial expressions should be limited for three to six weeks while the brow assumes a new position. Because areas around the incisions and/or scalp may remain numb for several months, caution must be used with curling irons and hair dryers. Ultra violet light may darken maturing scars, so care should be taken to protect them from the sun.

Since nothing heals symmetrically or suddenly, the best results can be expected from three to six months after surgery. As with all cosmetic surgeries, the best outcome is achieved by conscientiously following instructions.

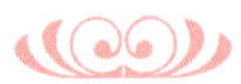

MID FACELIFT
(Mid Face Suspension)

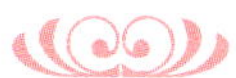

Understanding mid facelift

The goal of the mid facelift is to elevate and tighten the soft tissue of the cheek area. A secondary goal is to restore the lower eyelid and cheek region to a more youthful form. These goals are accomplished by lifting the fallen soft tissue on top of the nasolabial fold (fold or crease between the nostril, lip and cheek) and by reducing the hollowness between the lower eyelids and middle of the cheeks.

A youthful face has fullness in its central portion. During the third to fourth decade of life, this region may begin to droop and lose volume. Part of this drooping is a result of the sagging fat pads of the face or loss of facial fat. Sun damage, loss of skin elasticity and other changes can also hasten the gaunt or uneven look seen in many people over the age of 40.

When performed correctly, a mid facelift will result in a more natural, noticeable improvement. For younger patients, the mid facelift is a way to restore a more youthful contour without more extensive surgery. For older patients, the mid facelift is often performed with other procedures such as facelift, eyelid surgery, fat transfer and brow or forehead lift.

Understanding the procedure

The mid facelift is performed as an outpatient procedure with general anesthesia or local anesthesia and I.V. sedation. Dr. English places a small incision in the hair-bearing area above each ear. An additional incision is made inside the mouth on the underside of the upper lip. Instruments are introduced through the incisions to lift the soft tissues off the cheekbones so they can be elevated and repositioned upward.
A device is inserted to ensure proper placement of the soft tissues. The body absorbs this device in four to six months. The incisions in the mouth are closed with absorbable sutures to avoid the need for removal. Since the incisions are located in the hair and within the mouth, there is no significant visible scarring. It typically takes between thirty to sixty days for the swelling of the repositioned tissue over the cheekbones to subside.

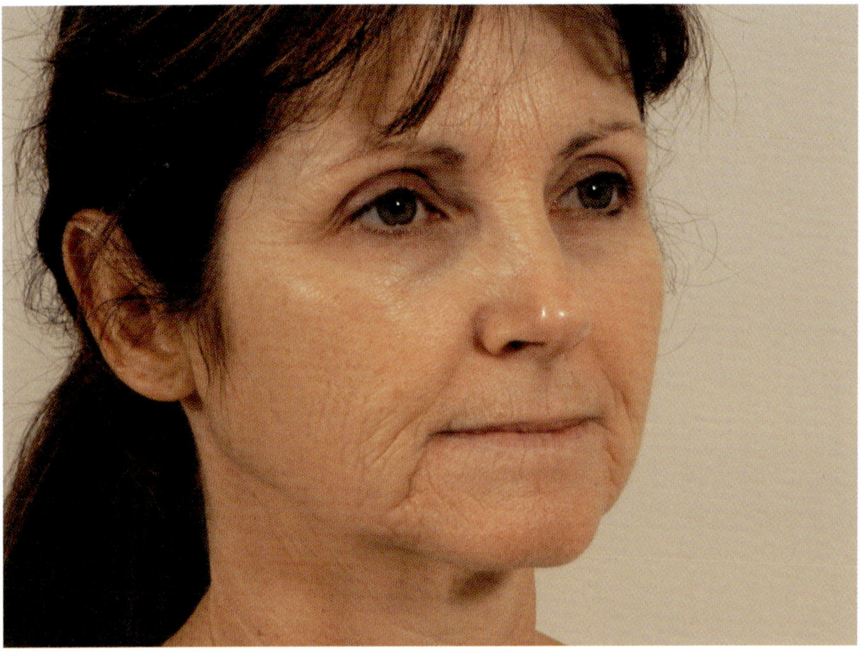

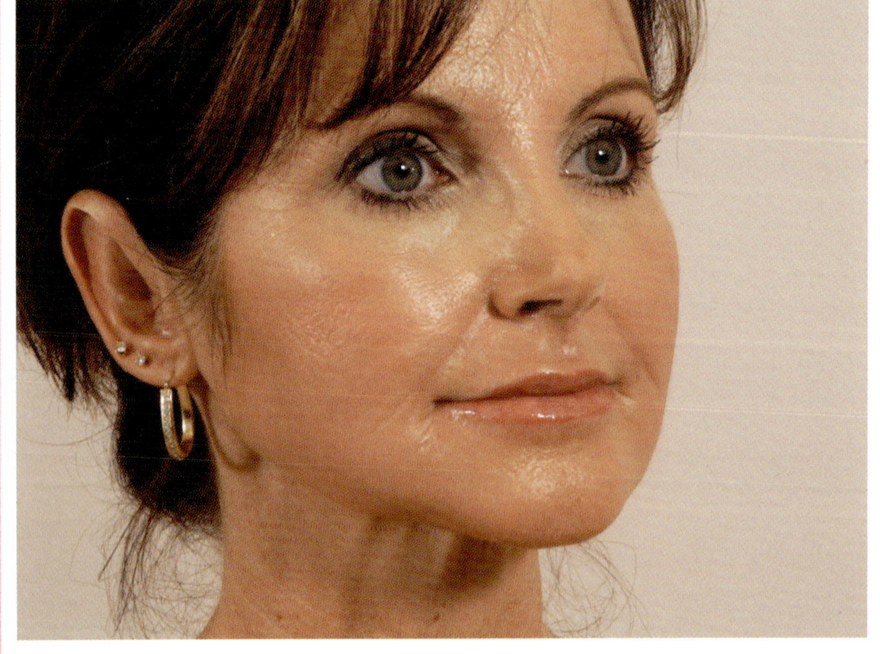

Understanding the recovery

Immediately following the surgery, the patient may experience some temporary swelling and bruising in the mid-face area. It is important to rest and sleep in an elevated position for at least two weeks following the procedure in order to minimize any swelling and bruising.

Patients experience mild to moderate discomfort that can be controlled with prescription medications. Chewing is limited for seven to ten days and a liquid or soft food diet is required during this time period. Activities such as heavy lifting and bending are limited for several days and facial expressions are also restricted. Pressure to the cheek areas should be avoided for four to six weeks following the procedure. Although the cheek areas are swollen and tender for a few weeks, recovery is usually rapid. Most patients return to work in a few days.

Numbness may occur as a result of stretching the nerve but will resolve as the swelling subsides. A wry smile, though uncommon, is another issue involving the facial muscles that resolves as the tissue heals.

NOSE SURGERY
(Rhinoplasty)

Understanding nose surgery

Nose surgery or rhinoplasty is performed to change the size and/or shape of the nose. This reshaping is accomplished by carefully removing or rearranging underlying bone or cartilage.

Most cosmetic nose surgeries are performed because the patient desires an improved appearance. However, the surgery is frequently requested to repair injuries, to correct breathing problems or to minimize the increasing disfigurement of the nose that occurs as an individual ages.

The appropriate age for nose surgery depends on many factors. For children, cosmetic nose surgery should be delayed until facial development approaches maturity. This level of maturity is usually around the age of 16 for girls and 18 for boys. However, nose surgery may be performed at a younger age if a severe breathing problem is present. There is no upper age limit for nose surgery. Patients in their sixties and seventies elect to have this procedure with good results.

Since the nose is usually the most defining characteristic of the face, a slight alteration can result in a more pleasing look that compliments other facial features. Technical refinements in surgical procedures have allowed consistently better results, however, patients must recognize that the goal of the surgery is improvement, not perfection.

During a consultation, Dr. English assesses the patient's age, height, skin thickness, ethnic background and shape of other features such as the forehead, eyes and chin. Nose surgery is as much artistic in nature as it is technical, so the surgeon should strive to make each patient's nose fit his or her face. The goal is a natural looking nose rather than one that appears to have been surgically altered. It is frequently necessary to correct a receding or protruding chin at the same time nose surgery is performed to provide harmony of the facial features.

Understanding the procedure

Nose surgery is performed as an outpatient procedure using general anesthesia or

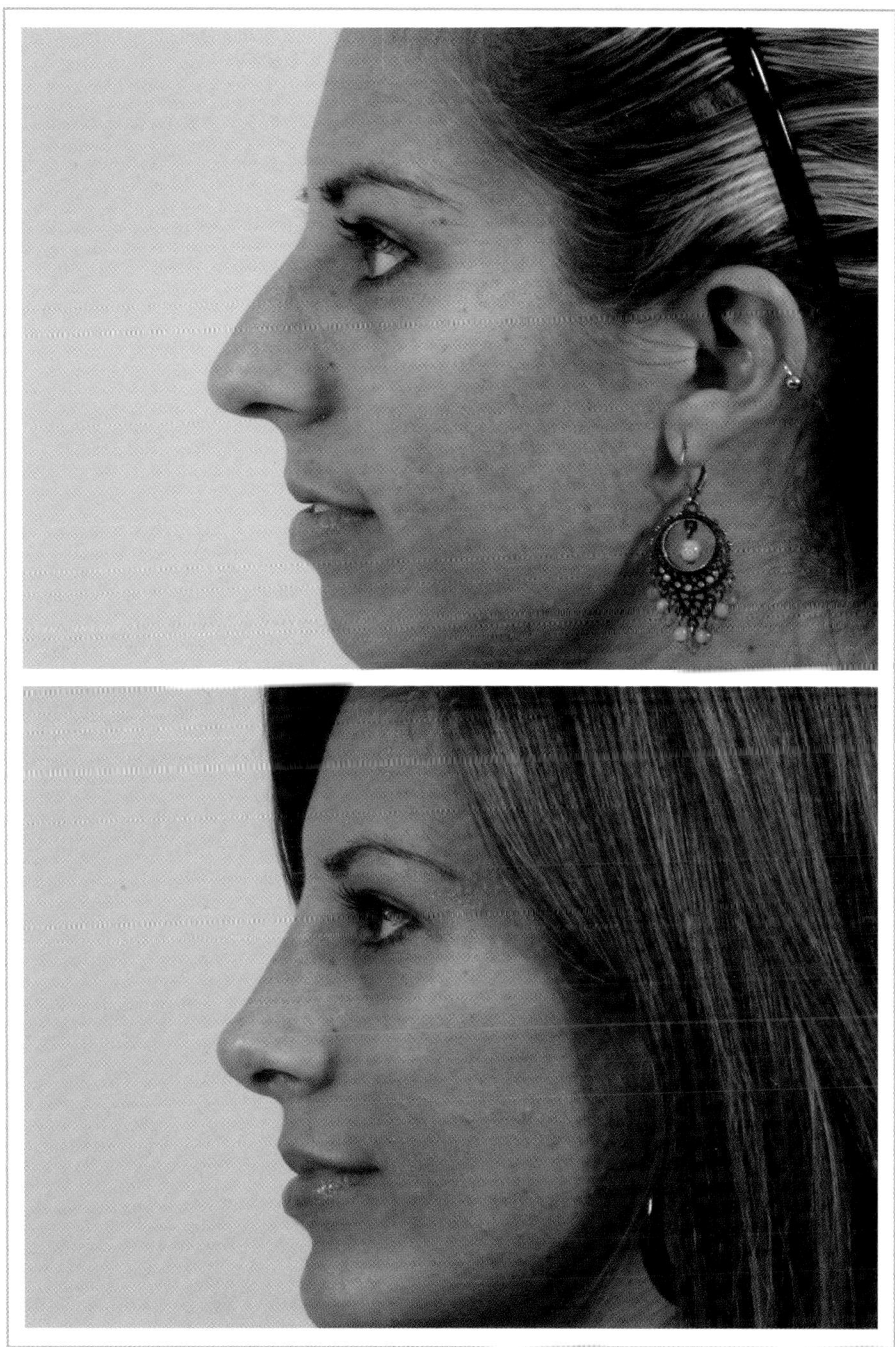

local anesthesia with I.V. sedation. Incisions are usually made inside the nose where they will not be visible. In some cases, an incision is made in the area of the skin separating the nostrils and/or at the base of the each nostril if narrowing the base of the nose is part of the procedure. Very fine, absorbable sutures are used to close the incisions. The sutures dissolve on their own usually leaving an imperceptible scar.

At the completion of the surgery, a protective splint is placed on the outside of the nose and a small amount of soft absorbent material is placed inside the nose to maintain stability. The splint and absorbent material are removed six days after the surgery.

Understanding the recovery

Swelling from the surgery usually peaks within 72 hours. Although most of the swelling resolves quickly, some lasts for several months. Bruising may develop in the face, particularly around the eyes, but usually resolves in three to six weeks. The patient may also experience nasal congestion due to swelling which may last four to twelve weeks. Numbness or tenderness may occur in the nasal tip or upper lip and may continue for six months to a year.

Some activities are limited during the weeks following the procedure to allow optimal healing of the nose. Exposure to the sun, physical exertion and risk of injury must be avoided. Forceful coughing, sneezing, blowing the nose or sniffing should also be avoided for the first few weeks. Contact lenses should not be worn for three to seven days after the procedure. Eyeglasses or sunglasses must be avoided for a minimum of six weeks to three months to prevent pressure on the nose as it heals.

Since resolution of the swelling may be asymmetrical, the final result may not be seen for months. In general, the appearance of the nose continues to improve for a year or more after surgery. It is particularly important to follow instructions after nose surgery to ensure the best result.

SKIN RESURFACING
(Chemical Peel, Dermabrasion and Laser)

Understanding skin resurfacing

Skin resurfacing removes the outer layers of the skin on the face to reduce and/or eliminate lines, wrinkles and mild to moderate scars. These procedures stimulate new skin growth, resulting in a fresher, more youthful appearance. Skin resurfacing is a time consuming, frustrating and anxiety producing experience, however, it can often produce some of the best results accomplished by cosmetic procedures. Chemicals, special surgical equipment and/or lasers are used for these procedures.

CHEMICAL PEEL: A chemical peel involves the application of a chemical solution to the skin of the face. The solution causes the surface layers of skin to peel away, leaving a newly regenerated skin that is usually smoother and less wrinkled. A chemical peel reduces or eliminates superficial as well as deeper lines in the facial skin. It is also helpful in reducing or removing freckles, age spots and splotching caused by birth control pills or pregnancy. The depth of a chemical peel is controlled by the amount and type of solution used by the surgeon as well as the application process.

DERMABRASION: When the skin has an uneven texture that results from acne or previous injuries, dermabrasion may provide improvement. The process of dermabrasion is similar to sanding an irregularity from any surface such as a wooden board. The more elevated areas of skin are smoothed down to diminish the high-low variations that cast shadows when light strikes the face. Also as the skin heals, the lower areas of the skin surface tend to migrate upward so as not to look as deep. Because the skin of the face is fairly thick, dermabrasion can be performed in all facial areas except the eyelids.

LASER: State of the art skin resurfacing is performed using a special beam of light energy that is absorbed by the skin and surrounding tissues. The laser pulse reduces or removes wrinkles and lines around the cheeks, eyes, forehead and mouth. This technology can also be used to treat some birthmarks, skin growths, facial "spider veins" and tattoos.

Understanding the procedure

Skin resurfacing is carried out under local anesthesia with I.V. sedation if the area to be treated is small. Resurfacing larger areas requires general anesthesia. When the skin resurfacing is completed, the patient leaves the facility with no dressings on the skin. Instead, the treated skin is covered with a thick coat of an emollient such as petroleum jelly. There is a fair amount of stinging in the resurfaced area for several hours afterward, but this is easily tolerated through the use of oral medication.

Understanding the recovery

Some degree of swelling follows skin resurfacing. The swelling is due to the tissue fluids brought into the area by the body to promote healing. When the fluids are no longer required, they are absorbed into the bloodstream. The patient can expect swelling to peak around 72 hours after the procedure. Most of the swelling is gone in two to three weeks.

The resurfaced skin takes six weeks to three to nine months to achieve the best results. The red coloration of the skin becomes pink and then regains a more normal color during the healing process. With some skin resurfacing procedures, the resurfaced areas may be lightened by approximately one-half shade after six to nine months. While the skin is healing, it is thinner and more sensitive. The "new" skin must be kept moist and protected from the sun until it thickens over time.

The patient must be willing to accept the temporary swelling and discoloration that occurs following skin resurfacing. Most patients feel the inconvenience is a small price to pay for their cosmetic improvements.

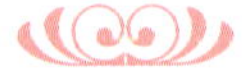

TUMMY TUCK
(Abdominoplasty)

Understanding tummy tuck

The purpose of having a tummy tuck is to remove excess soft tissue from the lower abdomen and/or to tighten the underlying muscles. This procedure is indicated when there is bulging due to abnormal stretching of the abdominal muscles and excess skin or fat. The extent of surgery depends on the amount of skin and fat as well as the laxity of the abdominal muscles. Symptoms such as low back pain, skin rashes and abdominal discomfort may be relieved as a result of the procedure.

Understanding the procedure

Surgery is carried out under general anesthesia. In some cases, the belly button is repositioned because of the amount of skin that is removed. Although hidden by clothing, a scar is unavoidable. The scar may widen and require surgical improvement at a later time, however, revision surgery is rare. Every effort is made to reduce the size of the scar and to make it as inconspicuous as possible through such methods as taping the incision post operatively. In spite of the incisional scar, most patients are enthusiastic about their results.

Understanding the recovery

Some patients run a low fever the first few days. Swelling around the incision can be moderate and peaks at 72 – 96 hours. As a general rule, 80% of the swelling is gone in four to six weeks and the remainder should resolve in four to six months. To minimize swelling, patients should rest and sleep in a reclining position for at least two weeks after surgery. It is important that patients sleep on their backs rather than their sides. Avoidance of salt in the diet also helps to prevent excess swelling. Hourly movement of the lower extremities helps to prevent leg swelling and blood clots.

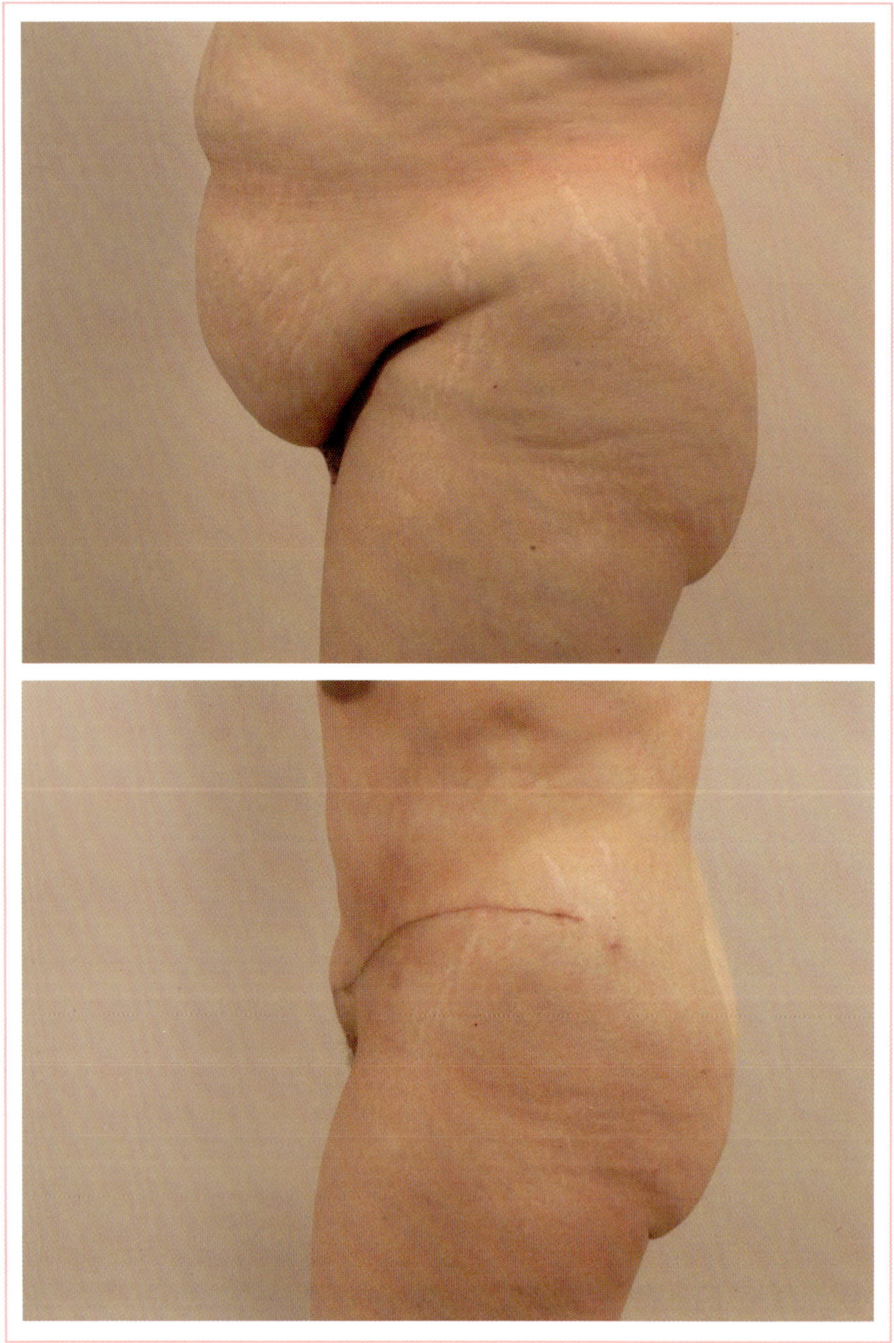

Bruising may occur in the surgical area following the procedure. If bruising develops, it should be much improved in two to four weeks. Some oozing along the incision may occur the first 24 to 72 hours after surgery. Areas of numbness, firmness and tenderness around the incision and under the skin are common. Normal feeling should return several months after surgery.

Lifestyle issues (for example smoking) or previous abdominal surgeries such as gallbladder, gastric by-pass, C-section or liposuction may delay healing. Since nothing heals symmetrically or suddenly, the best result will usually be achieved six to nine months following the procedure. The best outcomes result from following Dr. English's post-operative instructions and practicing good health habits.

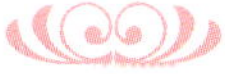

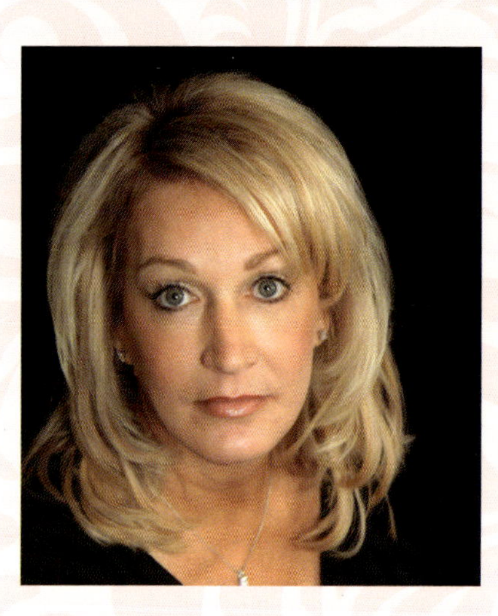

OTHER PROCEDURES

ARM LIFT *(Brachioplasty)*

The goal of arm lifting is to reduce and reshape the upper arm from the armpit to the elbow. The procedure is performed to reduce excess fat and skin and to improve the shape of the upper arm. Ideal candidates for arm lifting include healthy individuals with a normal body weight who have upper arm skin laxity.

The incision for arm lifting may be placed on either the inner part or the back of the upper arm. This placement is dependent on the patient's need and Dr. English's preference. The length of this incision depends upon the location and amount of excess tissue to be removed. The incision is closed with absorbable sutures that are under the skin and do not have to be removed. Although obscured initially by swelling and possible bruising, the improved shape and tone of the arm can be seen immediately following surgery

EAR SURGERY *(Otoplasty)*

Ear surgery is designed to reposition or "pin back" protruding ears. It is most commonly performed during childhood before the child begins school. While ear surgery is more commonly performed on children, an increasing number of adults want surgical help to have ears that are in harmony with the rest of the face. Even though only one ear may appear to protrude excessively, it is usually necessary to correct both in order to get the desired result

Ear surgery commonly takes from one to two hours depending on the complexity of the case. In most instances, the incisions made to reposition the ears are placed behind the ears. The resulting thin scars are usually inconspicuous.

HAIR RESTORATION

Hair restoration techniques are designed to redistribute the existing hairs on the head from the more dense areas to the thinner ones. During the preoperative consultation, the surgeon examines the hair and scalp to make a recommendation regarding the best procedure or combination of the following procedures:

Hair Transplants — Thin strips of hair bearing scalp are removed in order to prepare micro (1-2 hairs) and/or mini (2-4 hairs) grafts. These strips, from the back and sides of the head, are moved to areas where the hair is less dense. This technique transplants the roots of the hair so that once established, they produce hairs for as long as they would have at the original sites.

Scalp Reduction — Bald areas on the crown, top or back of the head are removed and the adjacent hair-bearing scalp is stretched over the area. Two or more procedures are usually required to achieve the desired result. These procedures are separated by several months to allow the scalp to soften and loosen.

Scalp Flaps — Areas of hair bearing scalp are transposed from the back and sides of the head to the areas where the hair is less dense. The use of scalp flaps allows for the transfer of a larger amount of hair which continues growing after it is transferred.

The placement of incisions is dependent upon the procedure that is being used. In all cases, the scars are generally quite acceptable because of their location and the coverage provided by adjacent hair.

HAND REJUVENATION

The purpose of hand rejuvenation is to help restore hands to a more youthful appearance. This area of the body is one of the first areas that age because the hands are constantly exposed to the environment. Common signs of aging include brown spots (age spots), wrinkling, loss of fatty tissue and loss of normal shape, volume and contour.

A range of treatments is available to enhance the appearance of hands: laser, chemical peels, fillers and fat transfer. During a consultation, Dr. English determines the treatment plan that best accomplishes the patient's goals. However, the prospective patient must be aware that hand rejuvenation is designed for improvement, not perfection.

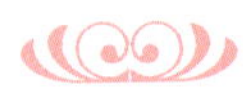

AFTERWORD

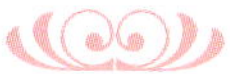

Stories. We all have them and in co-authoring this book, I was privileged to hear many. These stories of self-disclosure were told with introspection and honesty. Some were humorous; some were a bit sad. All were told with the sincere desire to help others who might have concerns or questions about cosmetic procedures. The women interviewed were from a variety of age groups and backgrounds. Some were just beginning adulthood while others qualified for the senior discount. They include secretaries, doctors, teachers and sales representatives. Most of the women had children. Some were busy with toddlers while others flashed pictures of grandkids. Many were happily married to supportive spouses. Some were divorced and happily single. The procedures they requested ran the gamut from breast surgery to facelift. Some of the women were very open about their cosmetic surgeries. Others preferred to be more private, disclosing their procedures only to a select group of friends and relatives.

Running through these varied narratives is a common thread, all of the women reported a boost in their self-image and confidence after surgery. Even a small change in appearance seemed to make a difference in how they felt about themselves. Most of them had a specific feature they didn't like that they had tried to alter or camouflage, often for many years. At some point, they chose to change the feature through surgery. This choice was never made in a frivolous or unthinking way. All of the women talked about the importance of having the procedures to please themselves—not others. Every woman was cautioned about expecting perfection or happiness as a result. Many emphasized the importance of carefully following the postoperative instructions. All wanted to send a message of encouragement to those who are considering a procedure(s) and all of them spoke about the importance of choosing a surgeon who is qualified. None of the women regretted her decision.

As a result of the interviews, I confronted my own thoughts, feelings and prejudices about cosmetic enhancement. I respect the women who choose the surgical option. I have equal respect for the women who don't. Because each person's life is unique, only the patient can decide what is best for her and how to begin the next chapter in her story.

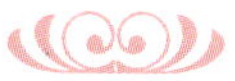